COMPENDIUM OF EARLY AMERICAN
FOLK REMEDIES RECEIPTS & ADVICE

COMPENDIUM OF EARLY AMERICAN
FOLK REMEDIES RECEIPTS & ADVICE

JON-ERIK SVENSSON

A BERKLEY WINDHOVER BOOK
published by
BERKLEY PUBLISHING CORPORATION

Copyright © 1977, by Jon-Erik Svensson

All rights reserved

Published by arrangement with the author's agent

All rights reserved which includes the right
to reproduce this book or portions thereof in
any form whatsoever. For information address

Sarah Jane Freymann
111 E. 85th Street
New York, N.Y. 10028

SBN 425-03367-8

BERKLEY WINDHOVER BOOKS are published by
Berkley Publishing Corporation
200 Madison Avenue
New York, N. Y. 10016

BERKLEY WINDHOVER BOOK ® TM 1062206

Printed in the United States of America

Berkley Windhover Edition, OCTOBER, 1977

Designed by Virginia M. Smith

For Sarah and Steve

Contents

PREFACE

MEDICINAL PREPARATIONS ... 1
"Feed a cold—starve a fever"

    Herbs & Herb Compounds ... 5
    "Nothing grows on this earth in vain"
        TEAS, TINCTURES, CURES & AIDS

    Medicinal Beverages ... 16
    "Don't drink the water till it has been boil'd"
        A PUNCH, AN ADE & SOME BITTERS

    Patent Medicines ... 26
    "Has cured others—will cure you!"
        AN ILLUSTRATED TOUR

BEVERAGES ... 47
"A Kind of Drink Called Rum"
        POSSETS, CORDIALS & PUNCHES
        LIQUORS

    Temperance Drinks ... 59
    "And on they came like a torrent"
        COFFEE, ICE, OR CAPILLAIRE?

FOODS   65
"A small hand will hold only 1-1/2 gills"

    Miscellaneous Rules For The Table   67
        MEAT & FISH DISHES
        VEGETABLES & SAUCES
        EGG & CHEESE DISHES

DESSERTS   95

    A Few General Rules for Cake Making & Baking
        CAKES, PUDDINGS, PIES & PRESERVES

TOILET & BEAUTY PREPARATIONS   115
"A perfectly safe and innocent employment"

        SOAPS, CREAMS & FACIALS

HOUSEHOLD TIPS   137

AN ODD & AN END   149

    A View of Women's Lib circa 1855
    Conversation

GLOSSARY OF TERMS & MEASURES   157

WHERE TO FIND & BUY INGREDIENTS   165

Preface

Interest is strong, and growing stronger every day, in returning to a more wholesome, natural and rewarding lifestyle. More and more people are baking their own bread, making cakes "from scratch," growing their own vegetables and herbs, delighting in the sense of accomplishment that comes from creating something with their own hands.

Of course, regressing to a totally self-sufficient ideal is unrealistic in the twentieth century, but there are a great many areas where we can benefit from the colonial heritage. I don't think rabies should be treated with vinegar, but I *do* think we should relish homemade biscuits rather than those mass-produced sponges that are referred to as "poppin' fresh."

Because it is my hobby to recapture what I feel are the good things of the past, I hope the reader will enjoy and use this book. Perhaps the advice given by Mrs. Abell in 1855 sums it up best. "Only those who, in their cares and toils, secure the most quiet, comfort, harmony and peace, who embrace in their schemes not only the pleasures of sense and physical enjoyment, but the moral and mental interests and pleasures, have best accomplished their duties, have won for themselves the most enviable reputation, and have most completely secured the well-being of earth's best paradise, Home."

Medicinal Preparations

"Feed a cold—starve a fever"

What is the difference between a cure and a remedy? What are the precise definitions of words like panacea and nostrum and drug? Who can say whether Doctor Merriwether's Miracle Tonic is a bit of quackery or honest-to-goodness folk medicine? Where, most of all, is the fine line that separates scientific from religious healing?

Ever since I became interested in colonial medicine I have found it difficult to separate myth and religion from medical reality. A perfect example of this is a cure for fever that was very popular in the early 1700s. It instructs you to cut an apple into three equal pieces. On the first piece you write "Father," on the second "Son," and on the third "Holy Ghost." Permitting the patient to eat nothing else, you are to give him one-third each day at precisely midnight. On the third day the receipt claims the fever will be gone.

I supposed this was one of those cures that depended wholly on faith, until it occurred to me that the logic behind it was sound: simply another form of "Feed a cold, starve a fever."

Sure, it adds mysticism and religion, but there's still a solid basis of accepted medical practice behind it.

Humor is another component of some of the cures. A bit of advice on "How To Cure A Cold" reads: "One tall silk hat, a four-poster bed, one bottle of brandy. To Be Taken As Follows—Put the tall silk hat on the right-hand post at the foot of the bed, lie down and arrange yourself comfortably, drink the brandy, and when you see a tall silk hat on the right *and* left bedposts you are cured."

Many early cures were based on observation of the animal kingdom. Instinctual behavior in animals was often turned to good use by man. For example, animals who have come out of hibernation in the early spring usually eat some greens first, often dandelions. Country people do the same, though they prepare the dandelions in all manner of concoctions from salads to wine. Yet both animal and man do so for the same reasons—modern science has found that dandelions act as a diuretic and are believed to cleanse the liver by stimulating the flow of bile.

However, man has been known to go to extremes when interpreting animal behavior. Most of us are aware that dogs take care of their wounds by licking them. The reason this works for them is that their rough tongues and saliva clean out whatever dirt is in the cut, and their saliva has antiseptic qualities. But the Romans assumed there was magic afoot here, so one of their sickroom specialties was a pie made of puppies' tongues!

Another example comes to us from an overzealous birdwatcher. He claimed that birds never caught colds and their preventative was demonstrated by the way they slept. Birds sleep with their heads tucked into their ruffled feathers, breathing warmed air. In the early Victorian period this was the justification for sleeping in overheated bedrooms. Unfortunately, the Victorians were wrong on two counts. First, birds *do* get colds; second, sleeping in cool rooms is much more salutary than sleeping in hot ones.

But for the most part colonial medicine was as valid as the knowledge of the time allowed. If, for example, you were stuck in the woods and hungry, the standard practice was to chew elm leaves. I've tried this, it works, and modern science still doesn't know why.

The colonials' belief that nothing grows in vain on this earth is being echoed in the large number of people planting and harvesting their own herbs. In colonial times just about every herb had some sort of medicinal or useful quality—pennyroyal and tansy, for example, were grown around every doorway to ward off ants and other insects and to make the house sweet-smelling. Flax was grown to make linen and its seeds were used in any number of medicines, from cough syrup to a paste for drawing out boils. Rhubarb was grown for use as a vegetable, a dessert, and as an ingredient in many medicinal preparations, especially "Stomick Soothers." Nasturtiums added colorful blossoms to the kitchen garden, leaves for salads, and roots for medicine.

Home medicine went into a slight decline when cities began to flourish and people were less isolated. This made it easier for families to buy patent medicines. Some of these medicines were guaranteed to do wondrous things like grow hair on bald heads, create third sets of teeth in toothless gums, and one—Doctor Grove's Chill Tonic—was guaranteed to make your children grow fat as pigs (a desirable condition at the time). Not content simply to make the claim, the label was adorned with a picture of a plump pig's body with a child's smiling head attached.

A favorite patent reducing pill turned out to contain tapeworm eggs. As soon as the unsuspecting dieter took the pill, the tapeworms began to grow in the intestine. The resulting weight loss was indeed phenomenal—until the person nearly wasted away from the parasite's voracious appetite. But then there was also an effective cure for "Deeply Seated Worms & Such." It recommended that the patient fast for three days, and on the third a steak be cooked in the same room with the sufferer. The steak was then to be held in front of his mouth. The cure claimed that the tapeworm would "leap from the Mouth of the Afflicted," famished and desperate to get at the steak. (I've not been able to verify this one!)

In the mid-1800s there was a patent medicine for everything—headache, biliousness, sour stomach, cancer, thunder humour, constipation, dyspepsia, horrid old sores, catarrh, deafness, colic, Summer Complaint, teething, inflammations, ulcers—the list is endless. This was a perfect period for the entrepreneur, and history records many who rose to fame, among them P.T. Barnum. From this era we have also received such terms as "snake oil salesman," "quack," and "medicine show." But lest you think the colonists were all dupes, the following from the *Farmer's Almanack,* 1809, should set things straight.

"From quack lawyers, quack doctors, quack preachers, mad dogs & yellow fever, good Lord, deliver us! This is my sincere prayer; let others do and say as they will. A respectable attorney is an advantage to a town, and ought to have the esteem of his fellow citizens; but a meddlesome pettifogger deserves the treatment of any other sneaking puppy that runs his nose into your closet. As for strolling preachers, 'O ye generation of Vipers' I would wear any evil far better than one of these intruding boobies! Yet how many forsake all business and pleasure that they may enjoy the ecstatic bliss of listening to their empty disgusting and blasphemous nonsense! The godly Mr. Bitemsilly's preach on—totally regardless of what the text of the sacred volume which says 'six days shalt thou labour and do thy work.'"

If you will not hear Experience, she will rap your knuckles.
(*Agricultural Notes,* 1811)

A work gives celebrity to a man's name, and after that his name gives celebrity to his works.
(*Allan's New England Almanack,* 1801)

We love those who admire us, more than those whom we admire.
(*Allan's New England Almanack,* 1801)

HERBS & HERB COMPOUNDS

"Nothing grows on this earth in vain"

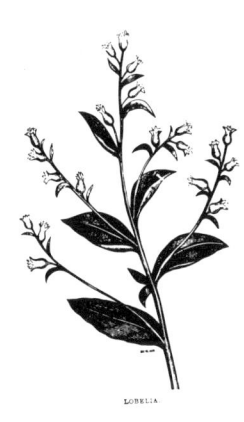
LOBELIA

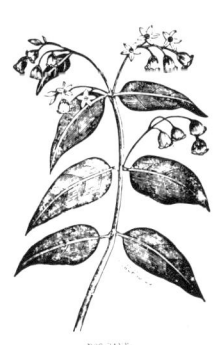

The use of plants in the cure and alleviation of bodily ills goes back as far as the history of man himself. The Old World had an enormous body of herbal knowledge, some of it dating back to the ancient Greeks. The immigrants to the New World brought this knowledge with them and soon combined it with the Indian's plant lore—thus the dawn of the American herbal pharmacopia.

Since the colonials had very few manufactured medicines at their disposal they had little choice but to take advantage of nature's bounty. This wasn't an easy task in a strange new land and there is much evidence to support the contention that the Mayflower's *passengers would have had a much greater casualty rate had it not been for the Indians showing them some of their native remedies. It's always seemed strange to me that instead of being remembered for this gesture, Powhattan won his niche in history for showing the Pilgrims how to fertilize corn with a fish.*

As life became more civilized and affluent, men started to collect books. Culpeper's Herbal *became the standard medicinal reference. Written by Nicholas Culpeper in 1640, its basic premise is that nothing grows on this earth in vain. Records show that it was in the collections of Franklin, Jefferson and Washington.*

Modern science has replaced many of the herbs, despite the fact that many possess useful and valuable properties. Many of the remedies in use in the 18th and 19th centuries have a solid basis in medical fact—digitalis is still used in the treatment of heart disease; mouldy bread poultices are "natural penicillins"; oil of clove still effectively comforts a toothache sufferer; puffball spores are still in use to stop massive bleeding—the list goes on and on.

We must remember that a good deal of these herbal medicines are more than just antique potions. Why use synthetic drugs when nature has provided in the fields and forests?

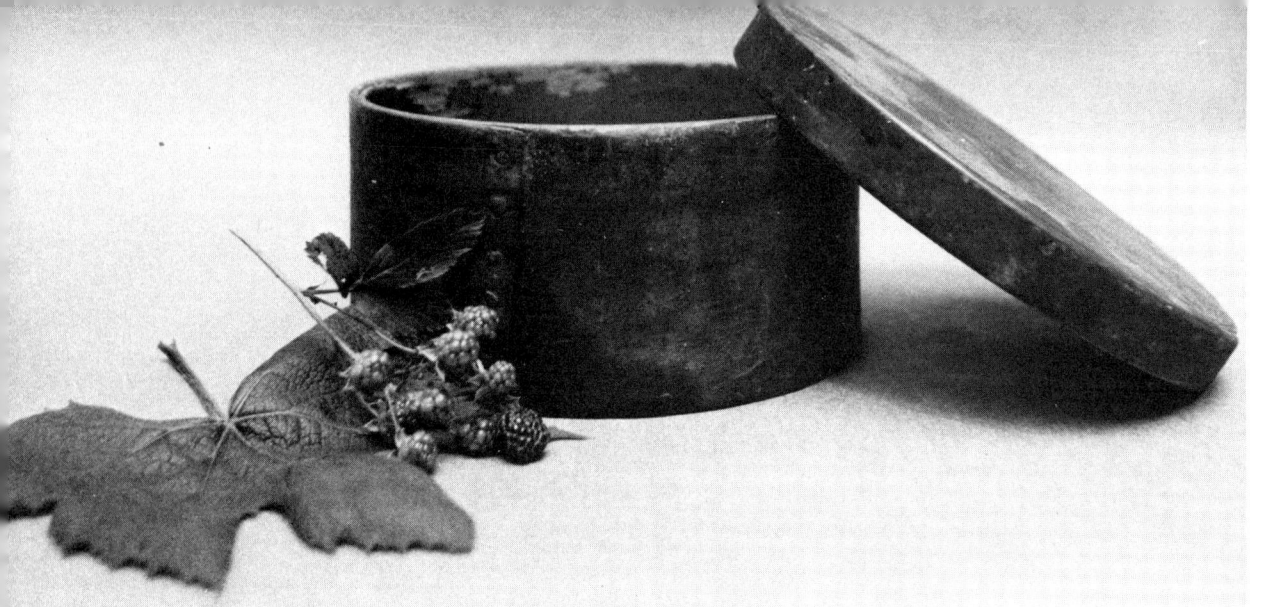

Perhaps Culpeper summed it up best in the introduction to his herbal. "What remains but that you labour to glorify God in your several places, and do good yourselves first by increasing your knowledge, and to your neighbors afterwards by helping their infirmities; some such, I hope, this nation is worthy of, and to all such I will be a friend during life, ready of my poor power to help...."

In colonial times herbal preparations, potpourris, conserve of roses, and many other homemade goods were given as gifts. They were acceptable and appreciated gifts the poor could give to the rich. Things haven't changed. If inflation has put the squeeze on your gift budget, don't despair. All it takes is a little talent and time plus some imagination. (You can even grow herbs on the windowsill!) And as you create the gift, you give yourself one, too—herbs are a part of life that everyone should take the opportunity to experience.

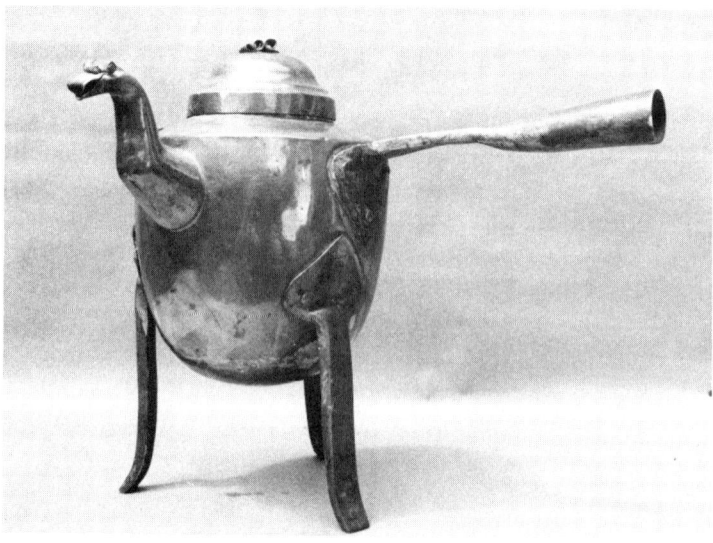

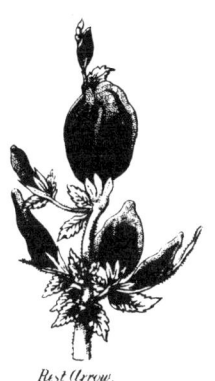
Rest Arrow.

Teas, Tinctures, Cures & Aids

Perhaps the simplest and most traditional method of using herbs medicinally is to brew them into a tea. The following method is suitable for just about any herb, if you like you can add some of your favorite brand of regular tea.

To Make Herb Tea: Steep the dried or fresh leaves or flowers in boiling water for at least five minutes. If steeping fails to bring out the flavor, the herbs can be boiled for a few minutes. If desired, sweeten with honey and lemon.

The making of a tea is an excellent method for extracting the medicinal properties from herb flowers and leaves, but it doesn't work very well when you're using hard materials such as bark, seeds, and roots. For these we must prepare what is called a "decoction."

To Make a Decoction: Boil one part of the herbal substance in ten to twenty parts of water for twenty minutes or more in a closed glass or enamel container. (I use one of those heavy enameled cast-iron Dutch ovens with a tight lid.) Strain and use.

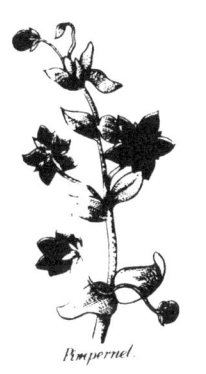
Pimpernel.

Teas and decoctions should be made as needed since they do not keep for more than a day. Any of the preparations containing alcohol will last almost indefinitely. To prepare an extract of any herb in alcohol, use the following method.

To Prepare a Tincture or Elixir of Herb: Add one to four ounces of the powdered herb (leaves, seeds, roots, flowers, or bark) to eight ounces of 150-proof gin. Steep for at least two weeks, shaking daily. Strain. Add four ounces of water and you have a tincture (50% alcohol); add another four ounces of water and you have an elixir (25% alcohol).

If you grow your own herbs or are able to purchase them fresh, you'll undoubtedly want to dry some of them for future use. The colonials hung them in bunches from the rafters over the fireplace where it was warm and dark, leaving them there until they were needed. In today's homes this is often impossible, so I've included the following method.

To Dry Herbs: Take a large jar (a dime-store fishbowl is perfect) and pack your herb in loosely. Stand in a sunny window until they are dry, usually in two or three days.

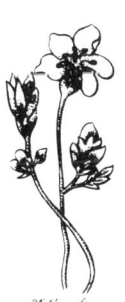
Its Saxifrage

Here in New England raspberry bushes grow wild along the roadsides, providing plenty of leaves for this receipt which is

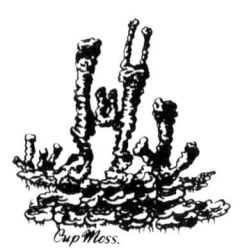
Cup Moss.

particularly good for stubborn coughs. It "rasps" violently on the way down your throat, but this feeling disappears within a minute and your cough is gone with the "rasp."

RASP BERRY CURE: Take one handful of Rasp Berry leaves and put to it a pint of water. Boil down to a quarter of a pint. Strain and add to it one Table Spoonful of Honey and two Tea Spoonfuls of Lemon Juice.

(*The Receipt Book of Anne Blencowe,* 1694)

Doctors still prescribe camomile compresses for eye-strain and puffy lids. This same receipt also makes an excellent hair rinse for blondes.

TO CURE WEAK EYES: Take a spoonful of Italian Camomile Flowers and boil them in a half pint of freshest milk, and when cool, dip a fine linen rag therein, and wash the eyes during the day for a week, and afterwards with clear water only for a few days. The eyes will feel cool & the sight become invigorated.

(*Beer's Almanac,* 1810)

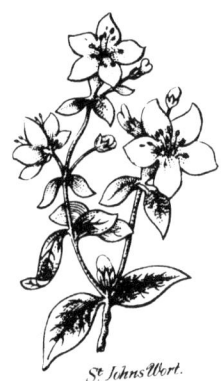
St Johns Wort.

It seems every old cookery book, almanack, and household advice book had a cure or two for warts. Here are some of my favorites—I've tried them all with varying degrees of success. Since warts often disappear with no treatment, it's hard to tell how well they work!

TO CURE WARTS: Rub them daily with a cut radish or with juice of marigold flowers, or rub them with a piece of raw meat.

(*The Farmer's Almanack,* 1798)

Rub them daily with the milky secretion from dandelions or milkweed, taking care not to spread the juice over any area other than the wart.

(*Success Magazine,* 1898)

Rub castor oil thoroughly into the wart every night and every morning until it disappears.

(an old manuscript receipt book)

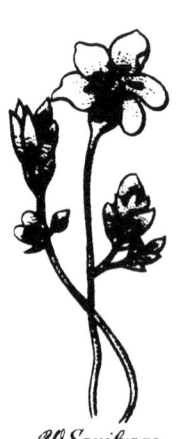
W. Saxifrage.

This piece caught my eye at a tag sale. All that was left of the original book were ten tattered pages, and this was one of the receipts. Today we call Indian hemp "marijuana."

NOTES ON INDIAN HEMP: Indian Hemp is a narcotic, anodyne and antispasmodic. It has been successfully employed in gout, neuralgia, rheumitism, locked jaw, convulsions, chorea, hysteria and uterine hemmorhage; but it is chiefly valuable as an invigorator of the mind and body. Its exhilarating qualities are unequalled and it is a certain restorative in low mental conditions as well as in cases of extreme debility and emaciation. In such cases

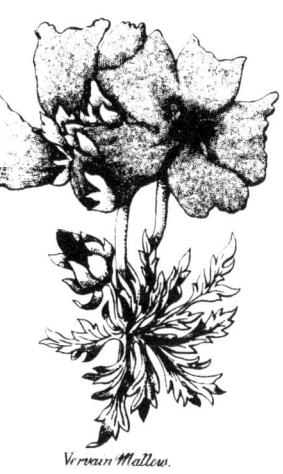
Vervain Mallow.

it may be regarded as a real rejuvenator. It should be taken by the advice of one experienced in its uses in order that its merits may be properly and fairly experienced. As this is a very powerful drug and poisonous in overdoses, I would advise all readers to use it only with the advice of an experienced physician. A teaspoonful of the herb to a pint of boiling water; a teaspoonful two to four times a day, cold.

(ca. 1890)

I usually don't get drunk, but last year at a Christmas party I did. The following morning I thought I was dying. Seizing the opportunity to try out some of the old "day-after remedies," I tried the following. It worked wonders, and the best part was that there wasn't any medicinal taste. The following cure has since been used with great results by many of my friends.

HANGOVER CURE: Arrange yourself comfortably in a quiet, darkened room. If there is still any problem with vomiting, put a few drops of clove oil on a sugar cube and suck on it for a few minutes. Next, chew a piece of parsley which will rid your mouth of the taste of the clove oil (and incidentally is considered a cure for a hangover by itself). Next, take a cup of camomile tea—lukewarm, *not hot,* sweetened with honey. About half an hour later take a teaspoonful or two of plain honey and continue to take another one or two teaspoonfuls every half hour for two or three hours. If you feel you must take aspirin, please don't take it before you've had the tea as aspirin tends to upset your already furious stomach.

(a combination of 18th & 19th century receipts)

I'm always amused when I run across this type of "guaranteed" cure in the old receipt books or newspapers. I really don't have the right to scoff, though—I fortunately have never found anyone in need of it.

TO CURE PARALYSIS: Place a teaspoonful of hops into a pint of boiling water. Strain thoroughly and let it cool and drink a cupful during the daytime.

(Miss Annie N.L., 1874)

Here is another rather strange cure. Whether based on faith or fact, the man who passed it on to us sure believed in it.

TO CURE BOILS AND PIMPLES: I am an old trapper and have received the following formula from an old Indian. It has cured me of boils. I used to be afflicted with these boils every year. At times I would have from one to fourteen at a time. Take the inner bark of

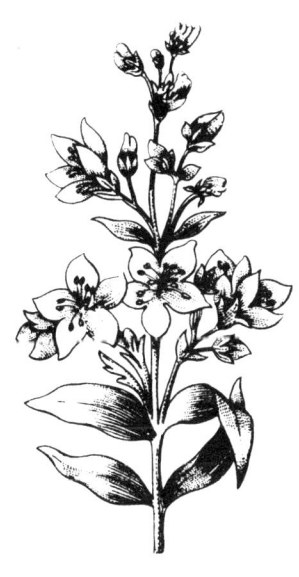
Yellow Loosestrife.

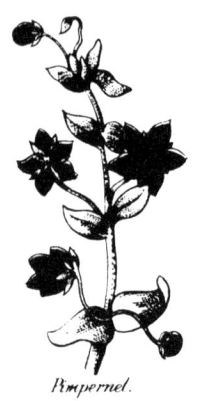

Pimpernel.

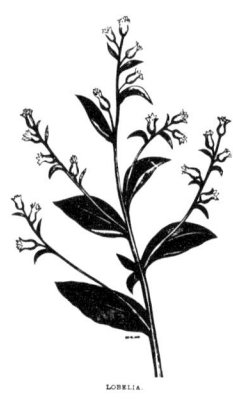

LOBELIA.

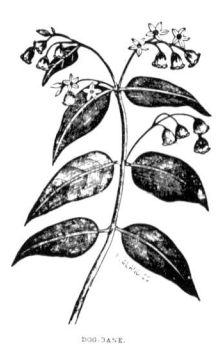

DOGBANE.

the birch, about a teacupful of the bark to a quart of water. Boil a few minutes. Drink in place of water.

(*Allan's New England Almanack*, 1828)

I found this gem hand-copied in a journal written in 1800, then ran across the original in a reproduction of *The Book Of Simples* printed in 1650. Whenever I find a formula for improving the head and memory, I *always* try it. In this case I wasn't able to decide whether it improved anything but my spirits—it definitely *is* a great cologne!

EMPEROR CHARLESES WATER: When roses are blown, take a quart of good aquavitae in a glass with a narrow neck and when the roses are half-blown take a handful of the leaves without seed, put them into the glass, and when the marjoram bloweth and the Apiastrum, take them a handful of their buds, chop them small and put them into the glass. Take also Cloves, Nutmegs, Cinnamon, Mace, Cardamum, of these an ounce and a half; bruise all these grossly and put in the glass and when the lavender and rosemary are blown add a handful of these flowers, also, shake them well together and stop it close; let it stand ten days in a hot sun; it must be used by annointing the temples and nostrells; it fortifieth and corraboreth the head and memory.

(*The Book Of Simples*, 1650)

The witch hazel available at the drugstore can't compare to this easily made extract. (And please don't forget that you can concoct your own private line of toiletries and medicinal preparations by using your imagination.) This particular receipt is improved by the addition of some thyme, rosemary, and a little lavender.

WITCH HAZEL EXTRACT FOR BRUISES: Soak a good handful of witch hazel leaves and twigs in 2 teacupfuls of the best rum. Shake daily for a fortnight and then filter through a fine cloth. Use this liquid on bruises, insect bites and as a generally soothing lotion.

(*Household Advice*, 1868)

Roses have been used for everything from colognes to cold remedies. Out of all the rose recipes I've tried, this is my favorite. Not only is it a soothing liquid for coughs but it makes your breakfast toast a real gourmet treat. (I've found that using rose petals in place of the leaves makes a much more interesting product.)

CONSERVE OF ROSES: Boil gently a pound of red rose leaves (well-picked, and with the nails cut off) in about a pint and a half (or a little more, as by discretion you shall judge fit, after having done it once) of Spring water; till the water have drawn out all the Tincture

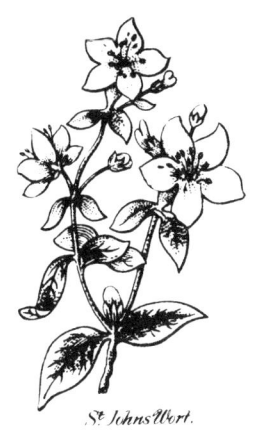
St. Johnswort.

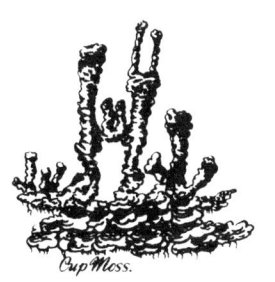
Cup Moss.

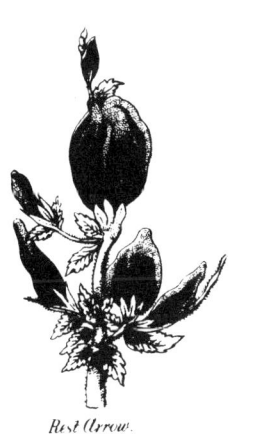
Rest Arrow.

of the Roses into itself, and the leaves be very tender, and look pale like Linnen; which may be in a good half hour, or an hour, keeping the pot covered while it boileth. Then pour the tinctured licour from the pale leaves (strain it out, pressing gently, so that you may have licour enough to dissolve your sugar) and set it upon the fire by itself to boil, putting into it a pound of pure double-refined Sugar in small Powder; which as soon as it is dissolved, put in it a second pound; then a third, lastly a fourth, so that you have four pound Sugar to every pound of Rose-leaves. Boil these four pounds of sugar with tincted Licour, till it be a high Syrup, very near a candy height (as high as it can be, not to flake or candy). Then put the pale Rose-leaves, into this high Syrup, as it yet standeth upon the fire, or immediately upon the taking it off the fire. But presently take it from the fire, and stir them exceeding well together, to mix them uniformly; then let them stand till they be cold; then pot them up. If you put your conserve into pots, whiles it is yet thoroughly warm, and leave them uncovered some days, putting them in the hot Sun or oven, there will grow a fine candy from the top, which will preserve the conserve without paper upon it, from moulding, till you break the candied crust, to take out some of the conserve.

The coulour will be red, and the taste excellent; and the whole very tender and soothing, and easie to digest in the stomick without clogging as does the ordinary conserve.

This conserve of Roses, besides being good for Colds and Coughs, and for the Lunges, is exceeding good for sharpness and heat of the Urine, and soreness of the Bladder, eaten much by itself, or drunk with Milk, or distilled water of Mallows, and Plantaine.

(*The Closet of Sir Kenhelm Digby,* 1669)

Potpourris and other sweet-smelling herbal preparations don't fit into the category of "Medicinal Preparations" by modern definition, but in colonial times noxious odors were considered disease-bearing and anything that masked them was considered an aid to health. Today there is nothing commercially available that even approaches the exquisite scent of a homemade potpourri, and now that we've reached the point, ecologically, where aerosols are being outlawed, consider a sweet-scented herbal preparation as a far superior replacement.

A POTPOURRI: Put into a large China jar the following ingredients in layers, with bay salt strewed between the layers; two pecks of damask roses part in bud and part full-blown; violets, orange-flowers and jasmine, a handful of each; orris roots sliced, benjamin

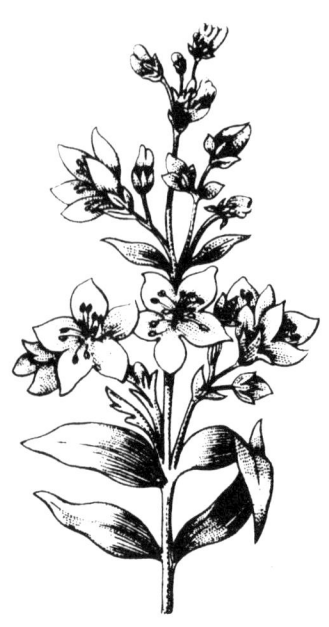

Yellow Loosestrife.

and storax, two ounces each; a quarter of an ounce of musk; a quarter of a pound of angelica root sliced; two handfuls of lavender flowers; half a handful of rosemary flowers; bay and laurel leaves, half a handful each; three Seville oranges stuck as full of cloves as possible, dried in a cool oven, and pounded; half a handful of marjoram; and two handfuls of balm of Gilead dried. Cover all quite close. When the pot is uncovered, the perfume is very fine.

(*Domestic Cookery,* 1834)

Another method of enjoying the scents of herbs and flowers originated in England—the Tussie-Mussie. It's simply a little nosegay made with a rosebud surrounded by leaves and flowers of various herbs you enjoy. They were originally used to ward off the plagues, but today I use them as favors at a dinner party or in place of a bow on a gift.

Still another method of using herbs as an air purifier and antiseptic was to burn them like incense on a dish containing a few glowing embers. Rosemary, lavender, and sage were particularly favored. Modern science has determined these herbs *do* have antiseptic qualities due to their essential oils. Again, our forefathers were on the right track.

> SWEET FUMIGATION: It is said the best plants to be cultivated for this purpose of disinfection are the cherry-laurel, clove and lavender, and the best herbs are mint and thyme. Narcissus and hyacinth are also recommended.
>
> (*Dicken's Home Notes,* 1896)

Some herbs not only killed germs, they got rid of bugs, too!

> HOW TO RID YOURSELF OF FLEAS: Spread around camomile flowers and soon you will notice that the fleas have left.
>
> (*MacKenzie's Herbal,* 1810)

Camphor is the traditional moth repellent, but there are other herbal compounds that do just as good a job with what is, at least to my taste, a much better smell.

> MOTH REPELLENT: Take one handful each of vetiver, rosemary and pennyroyal. Add to this five or six bruised bay leaves. Place in cloth bags where you store your clothing.
>
> (*The Christian Herald & Signs of Our Times,* 1871)

My apartment in Manhattan is more than occasionally visited by roaches. An old 18th century remedy for ants has worked wonders for me with my 20th century roaches that are seemingly immune to the

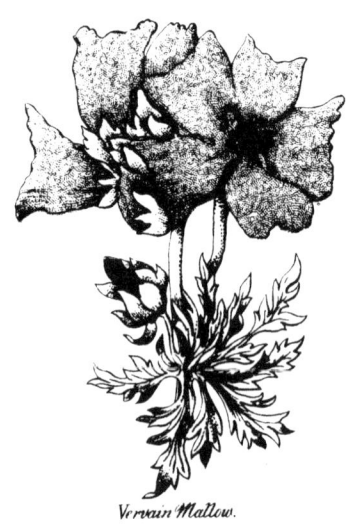

Vervain Mallow.

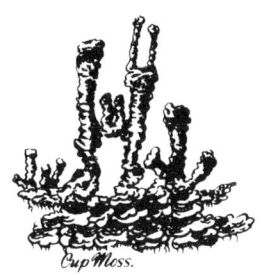
Cup Moss.

most sophisticated poisons. Just mix together equal amounts of oil of peppermint or spearmint with oil of pennyroyal and paint along baseboards, under sinks, etc. Believe me, it's really effective.

Another problem with life today is dealing with stress and insomnia. The colonials must have had problems of the same sort as they had a number of remedies meant to induce sleep and generally "improve the physick and constitution." There are several society doctors who are using the old herbal inhalants and sweet bags under the very up-to-date name of "Aroma Therapy," so as you enjoy these receipts feel confident that you're right-up-to-the-minute.

FOR A HEADACHE: Take a glass jar and half fill the jar with scented rose petals and lavender flowers. Pour white wine vinegar over until the jar is full. Close the jar tightly and place in the sun for about a week. Decant off the liquid and strain through a fine cloth. When needed for a headache place a clean cloth in some of this liquid which has been chilled and apply to your forehead.

(*Household Advice,* 1865)

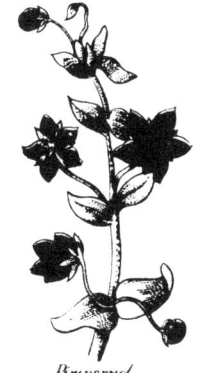
Pimpernel.

The most common use of sweet bags was to aid sleep. It amazes me that the overworked colonials had any problem with insomnia, but judging from the number of receipts for "Sleep Ayds" it seems they did. Here is one of my favorites, which is also very good for easing asthma.

A SLEEP PILLOW: Replace the feathers in a pillow with dried hops. If you see fit add some pine needles.

(*5,000 Receipts,* 1840)

This smells delicious and is extremely soothing when you're just too wound up to fall off to sleep.

A SIMPLE SLEEP AID: Take by weight three ounces of Rose petals, two ounces of Mint and half an ounce of powdered Clove. Mix together and place in a small cloth bag. Place it on your pillow when you retire and it will help you sleep.

(*Family Receipt Book,* 1830)

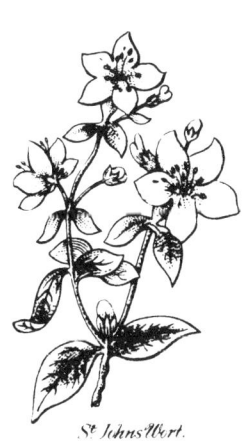
St. Johns Wort.

Admittedly, the ingredients for this receipt are difficult to accumulate, but if you're able to find all of them (or, for that matter, as many as you can) this oil is wonderfully effective.

A MOST PRECIOUS OINTMENT FOR ALL MANNER OF ACHES AND BRUISES; AND ALSO FOR THE REDNESS OF THE FACE: Take Violet, Primrose, Elder, Cowslip, leafs and flowers; Sage, Mugwort, Ragweed, white Lilies, St. Johnswort, Smallage, Marjoram,

13

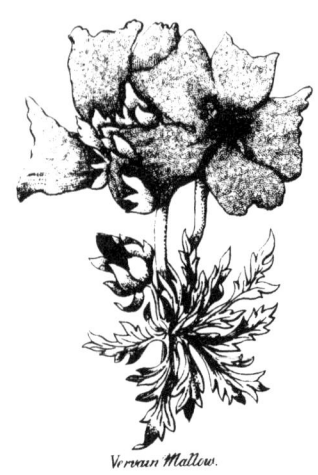
Vervain Mallow.

Lavender, Southernwood, Rosemary, Rose-leafs, Rue, Fetherfew, Tansie, Lovage, Mint, Camomile, Thyme, Dill, Clary, Oak of Jerusalem, Pennyroyal, Hysop, Balm, White Mint, Marygold, Peony-leafs, Bay-leafs, Saffron, each one handful. Stamp all these in a stone-mortar, as you get them put them into a pottle of Sallet Oyl, and so let them infuse there till you have all the rest together; for you cannot get them all at one time, but get them as fast as you can. Then put to them and the Oyl a quart of White Wine, and set it over the fire, and boyl it to the consumption of the Wine; then take it off and strain it; then put it into a glass and keep it for use. When you anoint any sore with this do it by the fireside, chafing it well in.

(*Receipts in Physicks,* 1668)

Syrup of Flowers was used as a flavoring, medicine, and a general restorative. The flowers most used were gillyflowers (carnations), roses, and violets. Use your imagination—I use the flowers from my herbs.

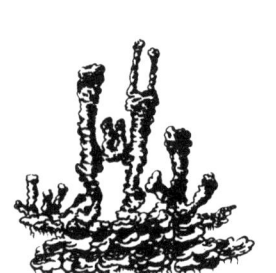
Cup Moss.

TO MAKE SYRUPS OF ANY FLOWERS: Clip your flowers and take their weight in sugar; then take a pot, and put a row of flowers and a strewing of sugar, till the pot is full; then put in two or three spoonfuls of the same syrup or spring water; tie a cloth on the top of the pot, put a tile on that, set your pot in a kettle of water over a gentle fire, and let it infuse till the strength is out of the flowers, which will be in four or five hours; then strain it through a flannel, and when it is cold bottle it up.

(*The Compleat Housewife,* 1736)

This is very effective at repelling moths. Because the scent is sweet and pleasant you won't need to air your winter clothes to get rid of the odor of commercial mothballs.

TO PREVENT MOTHS: Cloves, in coarse powder, one ounce; cassia, one ounce; lavender flowers, one ounce; lemon peel, one ounce. Mix and put them into little bags, and place them where the clothes are kept, or wrap the clothes around them. They will keep off insects.

(*Godey's Lady's Book,* May 1864)

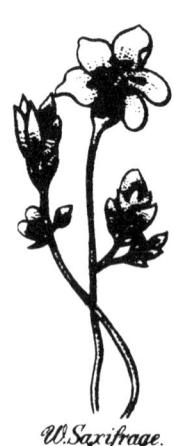
W. Saxifrage.

Celery is a very old and useful remedy for arthritis, and this method of brewing the seeds into a tea is perhaps the easiest way to derive its benefits.

CELERY SEED TEA: Take one ounce of celery seed and boil it well in one pint of water until it is wasted to half a pint. Strain and bottle.

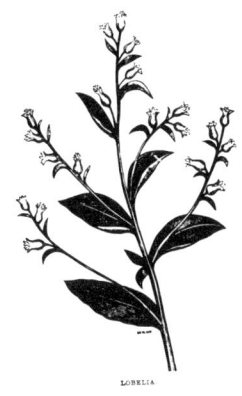

The dose is one teaspoonful a day. The effect is miraculous.

(*Household Discoveries*, 1868)

Coriander has been used for various ills, and all the old herbals attribute different qualities to it. This tea is very enjoyable iced with a slice of lemon.

CORIANDER WATER: Take a handful of Coriander seeds, break them, and put them into about a quart of water, and so let it stand, put in a quarter of a pound of sugar, and when your sugar is melted and the water well-taken the taste of the seeds, then strain it out through a cloth and drink it at your pleasure. You may do the same with Aniseeds.

(Giles Rose, 1682)

If you grow any fennel this is a wonderful way to preserve the liquorice flavor for enjoyment during the winter.

TO MAKE WHITE FENNEL: Take the branches of fennel, make them very clean, and lay them drying, and when they are dry take the white of an egg and a little orange-flower water, beat this well-together, and dip your Fennel into it and let it steep a little, then sprinkle fine sugar in powder over it, and lay it to dry before the fire upon a sheet of paper.

(*Receipts In Confectionary*, 1790)

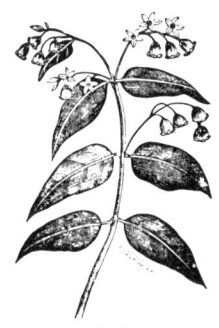

This works as well as anything I've ever tried on bee stings.

TO EASE THE STING OF A BEE OR WASP: Take a handful of Rue and crush it to extract the juice from the leaves. Apply it to any part hurt by the sting of a bee or wasp.

(*Helpful Advice*, 1801)

MEDICINAL BEVERAGES

"Don't drink the water till it has been boil'd"

Some of the most interesting receipts of the colonial era were for medicinal beverages. Even water sounds like an exotic elixir when described by Stearns in his herbal published in 1801. "... Wholesome, soft water... is an emollient, dilutant, dulcifying, refrigerating and diuretic... it assists digestion, renders the chyle fluid, softens & sweetens the animal fluids, dilutes thick humours, quenches thirst, abates acrimony, allays heat, cools fevers, removes rigidities, makes the parts flexible, excites urine, sweat and other necessary evacuations. It is the natural drink of all animals... it is of great utility both internally & externally in the cure of diseases; but it should not be drank, till it has been boil'd, as we observed before; nor should it be taken too warm, nor too cold."

The main ingredient in most medicinal beverages, however, was alcohol. It was one of the most powerful drugs at the colonials' disposal and no one can possibly estimate how many lives are owed to "Demon Rum." From a heart stimulant to an anasthetic for tooth extraction—indeed, the use of alcohol medicinally was so common we still have a number of jokes around about "Grampaw's Snake Bite Remedy."

One of the most common medicinal beverages was sulphur (brimstone) mixed into brandy or rum. Since sulphur was also in general use as an insecticide and fumigant, it staggers the imagination what its effects must have been when taken internally!

Many of the nonalcoholic remedies are still very much in evidence today. When was the last time your doctor told you to stay in bed and drink nothing but weak tea? The Seidleitz Powders of the 1800s are now marked under the names Brioschi and Alka-Seltzer. Buttermilk was used to build up an invalid's strength, and eggnog was prescribed for colds and queasy stomachs.

Again it becomes clear that lack of scientific knowledge didn't prevent the colonials from discovering many valid medicines by trial and error, some of which are still in widespread use today.

And again we can see things haven't changed much in two hundred years. Stearns recommends that rainwater be used when compounding medicinal preparations, but warns, "... it ought to be thin, clear, and void of any taste or smell. That water which falls in great towns and cities, is apt to be impregnated with the fumes of the city, & c., and therefore is not so good for use as that which falls in the country."

A Punch, An Ade, & Some Bitters

This is one of the most fabulous recipes for eggnog I've ever run across. It really is quite sublime made with milk "warm from the cow," but, lacking that, regular milk is fine, especially if you enrich it with a little heavy cream. It was drunk as a cold remedy and I'm sure it has just as much medicinal value if you let it cool to a reasonable drinking temperature.

MILK-PUNCH: One quart milk, warm from the Cow. Two glasses best sherry wine. Four tablespoonfuls powdered sugar. Four eggs, the yolks only, beaten light. Cinnamon and nutmeg to taste.

Bring the milk to the boiling point. Beat up the yolks and sugar together; add the wine; pour into a pitcher, and mix with it, stirring all the time, the boiling milk. Pour from one vessel to another six times, spice, and serve as soon as it can be swallow'd without scalding the throat. This is said to be an admirable remedy for a bad cold if taken in the first stages, just before going to bed at night.

(*Breakfast, Luncheon & Tea,* 1884)

My grandmother gave this to me often when I was a child, sweetened with large crystals of rock candy. I still use the same recipe today and this stuff's so good it even soothes a bad smoker's cough.

FLAXSEED LEMONADE: Pour one quart boiling water over four tablespoonfuls of whole flaxseed, and steep three hours. Strain and sweeten to taste, and add the juice of two lemons. Add a little more water if the liquid seems too thick. This is soothing in colds.

(*The Universal Cookery Book,* 1888)

A friend swears this was what he used to help him stop smoking. I asked a doctor and he said it could help if the person needed a source of nicotine while he was withdrawing from cigarettes. I only pass this

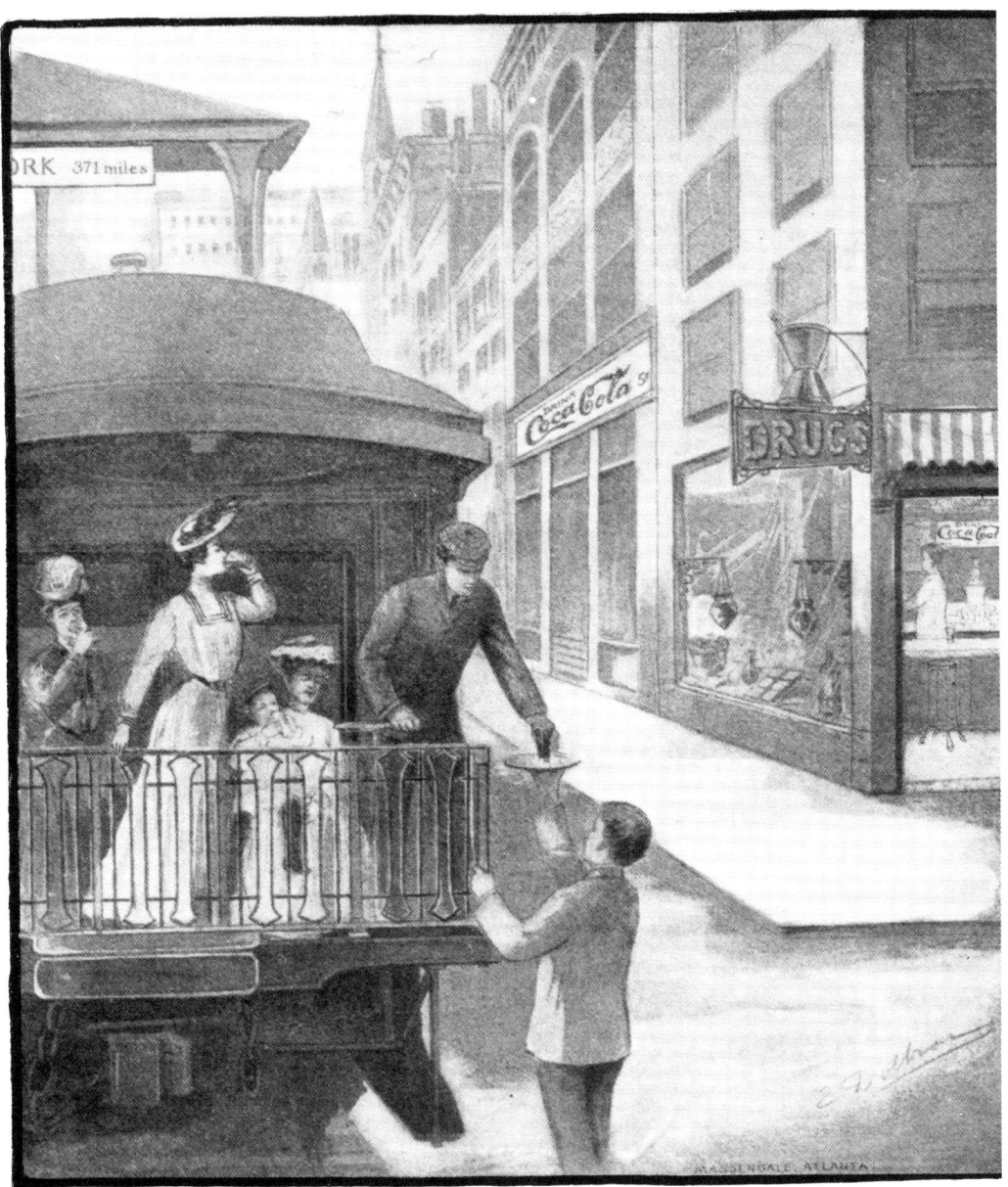

TRAVELERS' FATIGUE

— is delightfully relieved by a glass of Coca-Cola. Nothing so completely refreshes you after a hot, tiresome trip, or so brightens your faculties for the delights of sightseeing and travel.
Sold at all founts and carbonated in bottles 5¢.

information on—I really can't judge it one way or the other.

WINE OF TOBACCO: Take dried leaves of tobacco sliced, one ounce; Spanish white wine, one pound.

Macerate for seven days and filtrate through paper. We have already, under the article Nicotina in the Materia Medica, offered some observations upon its introduction into practice by Dr. Fowler, as a very useful remedy in the cure of dropsies and dysuries. From his treatise on the subject, the present formula is taken; and we may observe, that while in practice, we have frequently experienced from tobacco those good effects, for which Dr. Fowler recommends it, we are inclined to give the present formula the preference to every other which he has proposed.

Dose, thirty drops, gradually increased to sixty or eighty, twice a day.

(*Thacher's New Dispensatory,* 1813)

Saraspirilla has been considered a wonder drug since the 16th century when it was introduced into Europe from Mexico. In the 1700s it was thought that a decoction of the berries given to a newborn infant made him immune to all poisons. The colonials used it for just about every ailment from dizziness to syphilis.

A DRINK: Boil in a gallon of water two ounces of saraspirilla and two ounces of Spanish liquorice, until the water is reduced to three pints. This decoction may be taken at any time, even at meals; instead of water, ale, or porter; it is a good purifier of the blood, and slightly aperient.

(*Godey's Lady's Book,* October, 1859)

Root Beer was considered an excellent preventative against childhood illnesses. There *is* no doubt that it's one of the most healthful carbonated beverages you can drink, and it's sure to bring back memories for those of you who can remember what root beer tasted like before the advent of artificial flavorings. I suggest if you find you're interested in making your own bottled carbonated beverages that you invest in a bottle capping gadget. Believe me, tying corks down is very hit-and-miss and there's nothing more depressing than to find all your bottles have popped their corks.

ROOT BEER: For each gallon of water to be used, take hops, burdock, yellow dock, saraspirilla, dandelion, and spikenard roots, bruised, of each ½ ounce; boil about twenty minutes, and strain while hot, add eight or ten drops of oils of spruce and sassafras mixed in equal proportions, when cool enough not to scald your hand, put in two or three tablespoons of yeast; molasses two-thirds of a pint, or white sugar ½ pound gives it about the right sweetness.

Keep these proportions for as many gallons as you wish to make. You can use more or less of the roots to suit your taste after trying it; it is best to get the dry roots, or dig them and let them get dry, and of course you can add any other root known to possess medicinal properties desired in the beer. After all is mixed, let it stand in a jar with a cloth thrown over it, to work about two hours, then bottle and set in a cool place. This is a nice way to take alternatives, without taking medicine. And families ought to make it every Spring, and drink freely of it for several weeks, and thereby save, perhaps, several dollars in doctors' bills.

(Dr. Chase's Recipes, 1869)

There seemed to be great concern over the dangers of drinking cold liquids in hot weather. I don't know where this theory came from, but it certainly was taken with great seriousness.

TO PREVENT THE FATAL EFFECTS OF DRINKING COLD WATER, OR COLD LIQUORS OF ANY KIND IN WARM WEATHER:

1st.   Avoid drinking while you are warm: or,

2nd.   Drink only a small quantity at once, and let it remain a short time in your mouth before you swallow it: or,

3d.   Grasp the vessel out of which you are about to drink, (provided it is made of Glass, earthen ware, or metal) for a few minutes, with both your hands: for each of these substances conveys off a portion of the heat of the body, into the cold liquor; and thereby lessens the dangers which arise from the excessive heat of the body, and the coldness of the liquor, or:

4th.   Wash your hands and face and rinse your mouth well with cold water before you drink.

(Farmer's Almanack, 1806)

Not only were the colonials concerned about the temperature of their beverages, they were also very nationalistic, constantly discovering substitutes for imported goods. The reasons for this attitude are very understandable—foreign goods were expensive to ship to North America and when they finally arrived here they were inevitably taxed. Sadly, the American Revolution didn't solve the problems the patriots had demonstrated against at The Boston Tea Party.

NATIVE TEA: The infusion of good well-made meadow hay in boiling water, in the manner of tea, about three-quarters of an ounce for two or three persons, is a beverage for the fasting and evening reflection, as much superior to the dried leaves of China, as

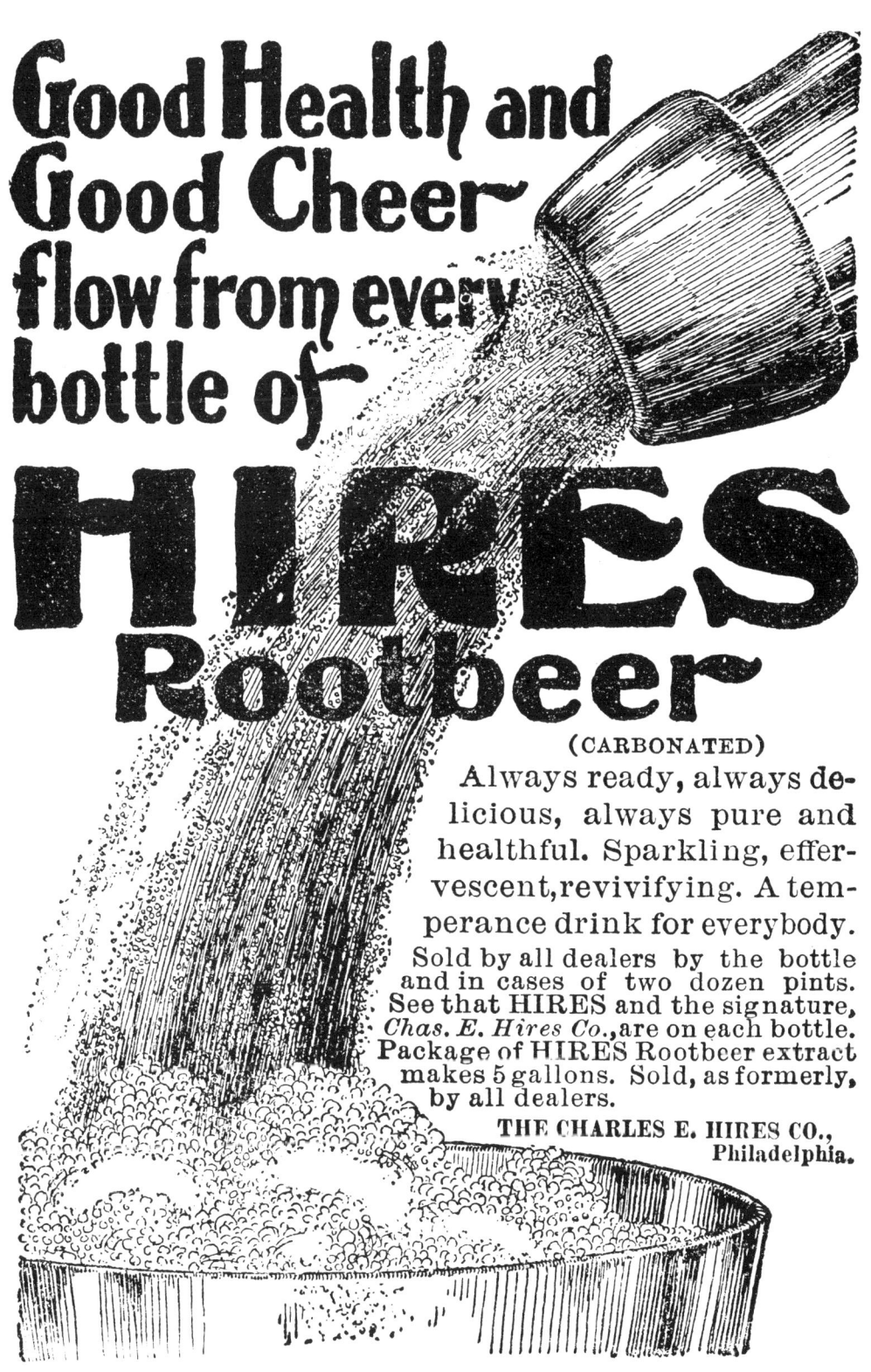

gold or silver are superior to copper and lead. This native tea is healthful as it is grateful to the palate; it is saccharine and aromatic, instead of bitter and empyreumatic; it is stimulating to the spirits in the morning, and composing to the nerves at night; it is antibilous, and acts with a mild, but sensible effect, at first, on all the secretions, promotes digestion and creates appetite.

(Mackenzie's 5,000 Receipts, 1829)

Not satisfied to simply state that a receipt was a good substitute, this one claimed to cure "inveterate headaches" at the same time!

GROUND IVY TEA: Make an infusion of ground ivy, which is very agreeable in flavor, especially if you add to it a drop or two of lemon juice. It is reported by many, that the habitual use of this herb will cure the most obstinate consumption. It is certainly a good pectoral, and when green is fragrant; if mixed with a few flowers of lavender, it makes a most agreeable liquor for summer use; and, if gathered at a proper time, has an agreeable taste to many, but wholesome to all, even when dry.

(Family Receipt Book, 1819)

Everything nature provided was put to good use. I've tried this one in lieu of Kaopectate and haven't really been able to decide if it's effective, but the flavor is so unusual (I like it a lot) it certainly could also be used as a general tonic.

CURE FOR DYSENTERY: A customer, every way disinterested, wishes through the means of your useful Almanac, to make known to the public, a remedy, which he is well authorised to say, has been found perfectly efficacious in curing the most inveterate fluxes of every kind, in the most desperate cases, after every other remedy proposed, had been tried in vain, viz. Dry large black bramble berries, when perfectly ripe (which in the summer season are to be had in plenty) over the fire in a frying pan, or in an oven on tin or iron sheets, until they are dry enough to grind in a coffee mill; when ground, put two ounces of the powder into a quart of good port or claret wine to which add two ounces of refined loaf sugar and a gill of water, which when mixed together, boil over a slow fire for about three-quarters of an hour, until it decreases to a gill, when cool, strain it through a thin clean rag. A small teacup full of this mixture for an adult, taken in the morning and evening, will effect a cure. A proportionate quantity (according to their age) will answer for children. This liquid, when so prepared, will keep good, if put into a bottle well corked and waxed, or the powder of the berries will retain its virtue for a long time, provided it be put into bottles and kept well corked until wanted.

(*Beer's Almanac,* 1800)

Rabies must have been a grave problem in colonial times as there are quite a number of cures given in the almanacs, cookery books and herbals. It strains the credibility of colonial medicine if you take everything literally—I'm rather sure that these people aren't giving us worthless cures; instead, my suspicion is that they considered just about every dog bite rabid, hence, many victims were cured of a disease they never had.

RECIPE TO CURE THE BITE OF A MAD DOG: A person not long since was severely bitten by one of these ferocious animals, and in a short time was seized with strong and violent symptoms of the Hydro Phobiae. A physician was called in, who prescribed for him, but by unfortunate accident and mistake, a large quantity of Vinegar was substituted in lieu of the prescription, which he patiently swallowed, and was recalled by it from the brink of the grave to health & life.

(*Allan's New England Almanack,* 1801)

Wine bitters were a very popular general medicine usually taken more as a preventative than a cure. Special racks were made to hold the necessary paraphernalia for wine bitters, and, judging from the great consumption of this mixture, it was used as regularly as we use aspirin today.

WINE BITTERS: Take balmony, bayberry, cassia buds, and bitter-root 8 oz., golden seal 12 oz., anise seed 4 oz., cloves 2 oz., cayenne 1 oz., brown sugar 3 lbs., pulverized and mixed; put 1 oz. of the powder steeped in hot water to a quart of the wine. These are said to be the celebrated wine bitters prepared by Dr. John Thomson. The wine bitters are a very pleasant restorative for debilitated people and convalescents. Very useful in dyspepsia, sick-headache, heart-burn, sinking, torpid feelings, and when-ever a tonic is required.

(*Book Of Health,* 1843)

This receipt yields a carbonated beverage very much like the British ginger beer. All the ingredients are healthful, even more so if you substitute honey for the sugar.

SPANISH GINGERETTE: To each gallon of water put 1 lb. of white sugar; 1/2 oz. best bruised ginger root; 1/4 oz. cream of tartar, and 2 lemons sliced. Directions: In making 5 gallons boil the ginger and lemons 10 minutes in 2 gals. of the water; the sugar and the cream of tartar to be dissolved in the cold water, and mix all, and add 1/2 pint of good yeast; let it ferment over night, strain and bottle in the morning.

This is a valuable recipe for a cooling and refreshing beverage; compounded of ingredients highly calculated to assist the stomach, and is recommended to persons suffering with Dyspepsia or Sick Headache.

It is much used in European countries, and persons having once tested its virtues will constantly use it as a common drink. And for saloons, or groceries, no temperance beverage will set it aside.

(*Dr. Chase's Recipes,* 1869)

If you like strawberries I'm sure you'll love this—it's incredible what a difference natural flavorings make. Don't be afraid—be the first in your neighborhood to make your own soft drinks!

ROYAL STRAWBERRY ACID: Take three pounds of ripe strawberries, two ounces of citric acid, and one quart of Spring water. Dissolve the acid in the water and pour it on the strawberries, and let them stand in a cool place twenty-four hours. Then drain the liquid off and pour it on to three pounds more of strawberries, and let it stand twenty-four hours. Then add to the liquid its own weight of sugar, boil it three or four minutes (in a porcelain-lined preserve kettle, lest metal affect the taste), and when cool, cork it in bottles lightly for three days, and then tight, and seal them. Keep it in a dry and cool place, where it will not freeze. It is very delicious for the sick, or the well.

(*Beecher's Receipt Book,* 1857)

Here's the original Geritol!

WINE OF IRON: Take of purified filings of iron, one ounce, Spanish white wine, sixteen ounces. Digest for a month, often shaking the vessel, and then filtrate.

This is merely a solution of tartarized iron in wine; for the iron is only dissolved in the wine by means of the super-tartrite of potass it contains. But a solution of a known proportion of tartarized iron in wine, will give a medicine of more equal powers, and may be made extemporaneously. The dose is from a drachm to half an ounce, twice or thrice a day in chlorotic cases.

(*Thacher's New Dispensatory,* 1813)

This tonic was taken to both cure and prevent every disease imaginable. I don't know what its real benefits are, but it tastes good.

GOOD ADVICE TO ALL PEOPLE TO MAKE A DRINK WHICH THEY

MAY DRINK AS THEY DRINK COFFEE, CHOCOLET AND TEA: Take a quart of spring water, and boil it till it wastes one third part, when you have so done, your water being boiling hot, put in twenty or thirty leaves of good Sage, and half the quantity of Rosemary, with fifteen or twenty grains of good Saffron, and let it infuse hot as before, for about a quarter of an hour close stopped; then pour it out clear from the Ingredients, drink it as hot as you can, taking about a quarter or a half pint of it at a time, sweetened with a little white sugar; and question not but the benefits you will receive will be far more and better this spring and hereafter than you have ever done by those liquors that so many commend; but the virtues of these plants are so universally known to be of such admirable Qualities, that I shall say of them that they are the best Plants that grow in this land, which is a climate and country which I may boldly say is so well furnished with Herbs and Plants which for Virtue and Goodness is not inferior to any country in the whole World, and these I have pitched upon are of its choicest Product.
(*The Receipt Book Of Henry Howard,* 1710)

I've tried both of these headache remedies, and the second one seems to help, or at least take your mind off it!
SICK HEADACHE: Take a tea-spoonful of powdered charcoal in molasses every morning, and wash it down with a little tea; or, drink half a glass of raw rum or gin, and drink freely of mayweed tea.

(*Family Physician,* 1840)

This works as well as any hiccough remedy I've ever tried.
HICCOUGH: Take five drops of the oil of amber in mint tea, every ten minutes, until they cease.

(*Helpful Remedies,* 1849)

Scientists have recently found that garlic is capable of killing certain viruses, so again the colonials were on the right track.
CHILL AND FEVER: Take three cents worth of garlic and half a pint of rye whiskey, put them in a bottle, and take a tablespoonful (for an adult) at night, on going to bed, if free from chill or fever,—if not, some time through the day. Previous to taking the above, take a dose of magnesia to cleanse the stomach. A few spoonsful will cure, followed as above.

(*The Mother's Book of Daily Duties,* 1855)

Patent Medicines

"Has cured others—will cure you!"

The term "Patent medicine" comes from England where the king often granted "Patents Of Royal Favor" to every trade imaginable—candle makers, soap makers, tailors—that served the royal family. The early colonials, loyal Englishmen to the core, favored those medicines which were endorsed by the royal family—the "Patents." The term has absolutely nothing to do with the United States Patent Office. Clearly, the last thing any Patent medicine maker would want to do was disclose the ingredients of his secret concoction. This, however, is a requirement for any product seeking a U.S. patent.

The Patent medicine era created a whole new breed of merchandiser. They learned all sorts of tricks, such as the fact that the public could be trained to ask for a particular brand of medicine, thus forcing a retailer to carry it. They also learned the value of advertising. Their goal was that every surface in the entire country be covered with an ad containing testimonials for their product. As large a bill as this seems to fill, a few of the more energetic promoters almost succeeded.

The use of narcotics in Patent medicines was so common around the period of the Civil War that drug addiction became known as the "Army Disease." The brilliant if unethical hucksters who manufactured these products had an ongoing business—they'd create an addict with one product and then "cure" it with another. This in turn would create its own new addiction which, of course, called for a new cure. Drug addicts were so common at the turn of the century that Sears, Roebuck & Company offered "Sear's Cure for The Opium & Morphine Habit."

However, the major reason Patent medicines came under such heavy attack, which culminated in The Pure Food & Drug Act of 1906, was that the advertising used by the Patent medicine promoters induced an ignorant public into treating themselves for medical *problems much too serious for self-treatment. One product, Kennedy's Medical Discovery, was guaranteed to "cure Horrid Old Sores of 40 years standing, Deep-Seated Ulcers, Inward Tumors, and every disease of the skin, except Thunder Humor, and Cancer that has taken root." How could a gullible public go wrong for $1.50 a bottle?*

Quacks, hucksters and dishonest men will always be with us, but with the passage of The Pure Food & Drug Act the Patent medicine era came to a halt. Sure, there are plenty of useless nostrums still on the shelves, but an unsuspecting mother no longer runs the risk of turning her six-month-old child into a morphine addict.

A physician examining a student as to his progress, asked him—"Should a man fall into a well forty-feet deep, and strike his head against one of the tools with which he had been digging, what would your course be if called in as surgeon?"
The Student replied, "I should advise them to let the man lie, and fill up the well."

(*The American Domestic Cook Book*, 1868)

Epitaph on John Foot: Here lies one Foot, whose death may thousands save:
For Death has got one Foot within the grave!

(*Beer's Almanac*, 1811)

An Illustrated Tour

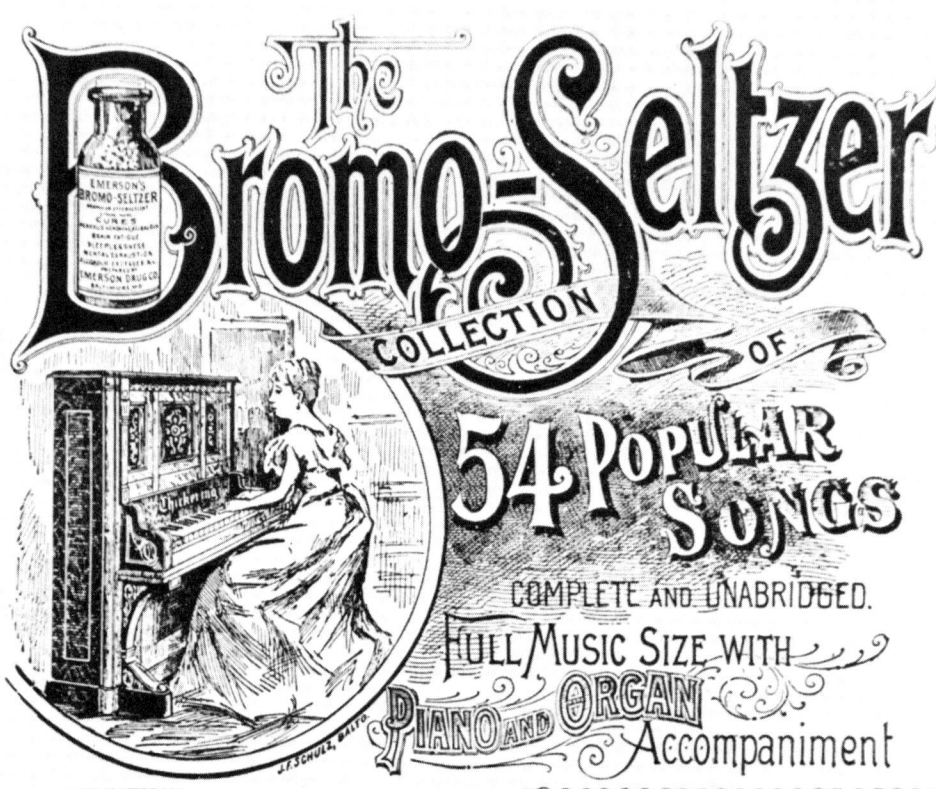

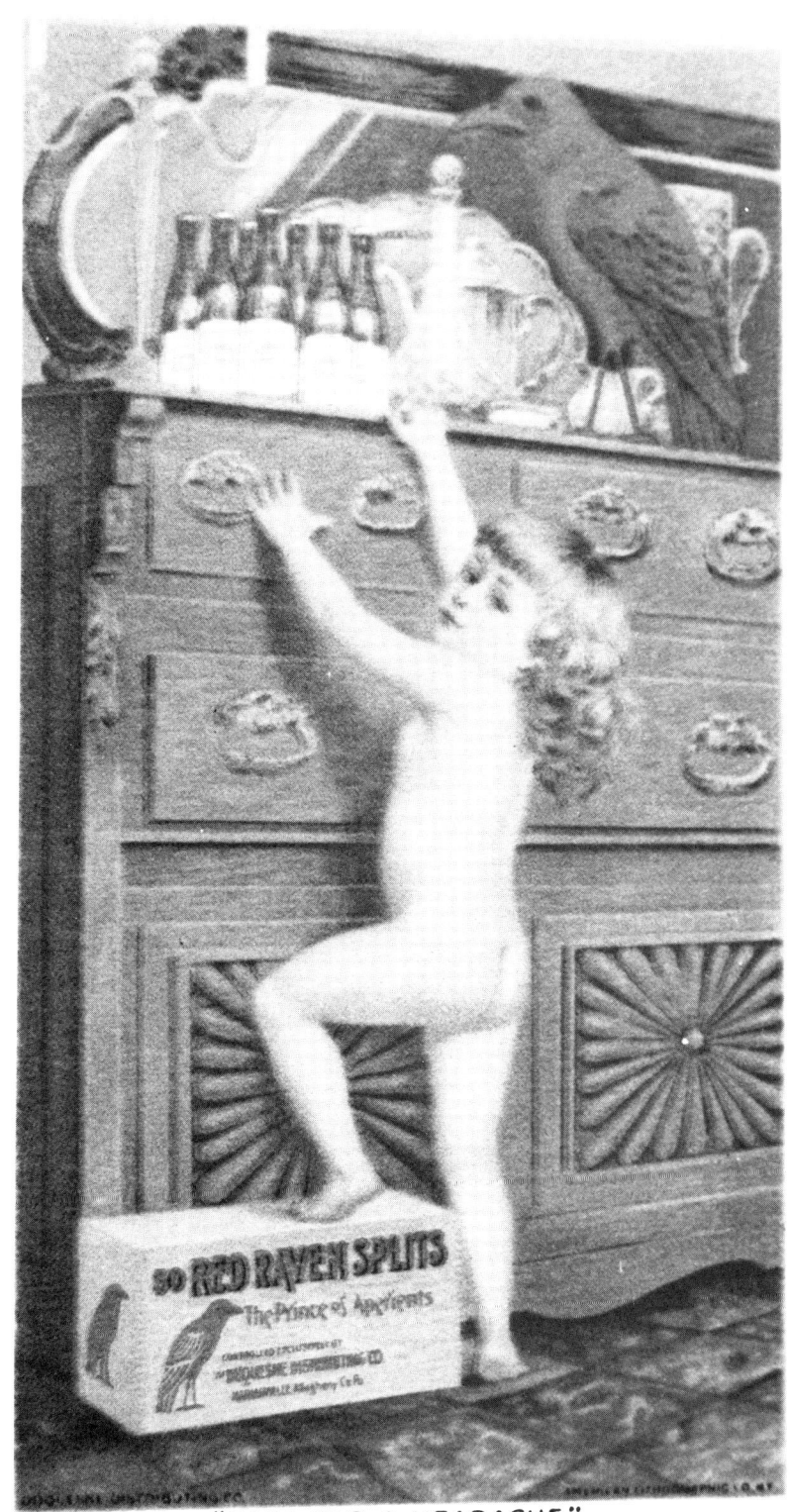

"PAPA HAS A HEADACHE"

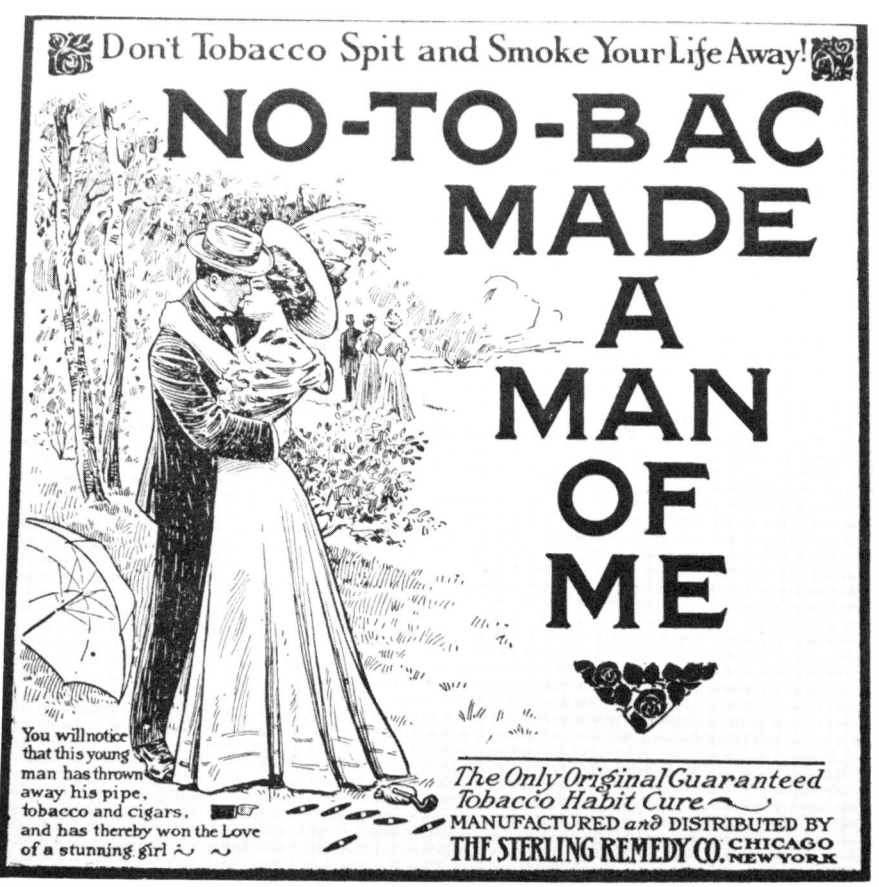

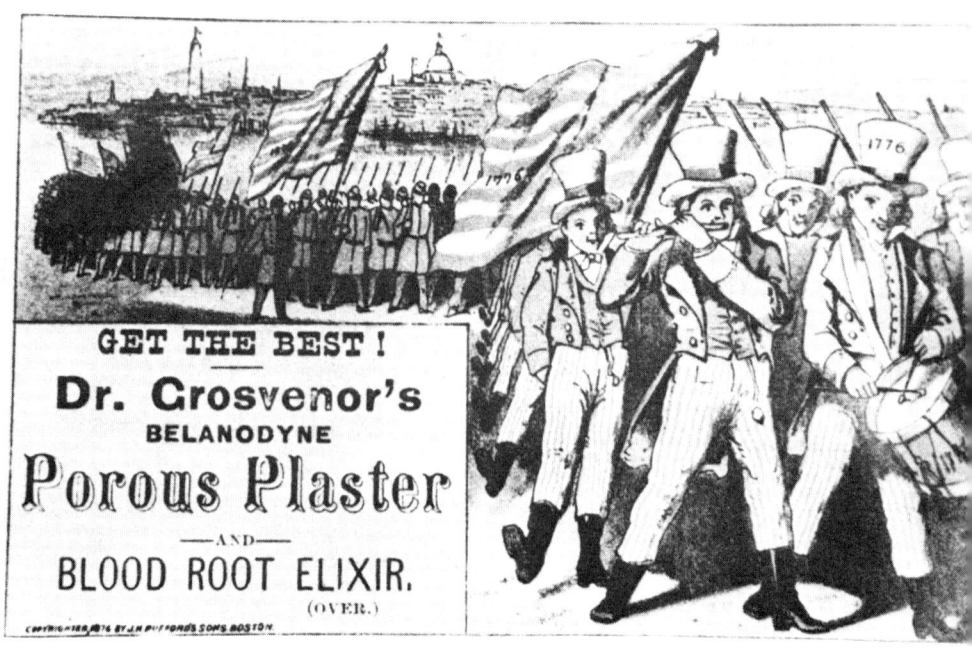

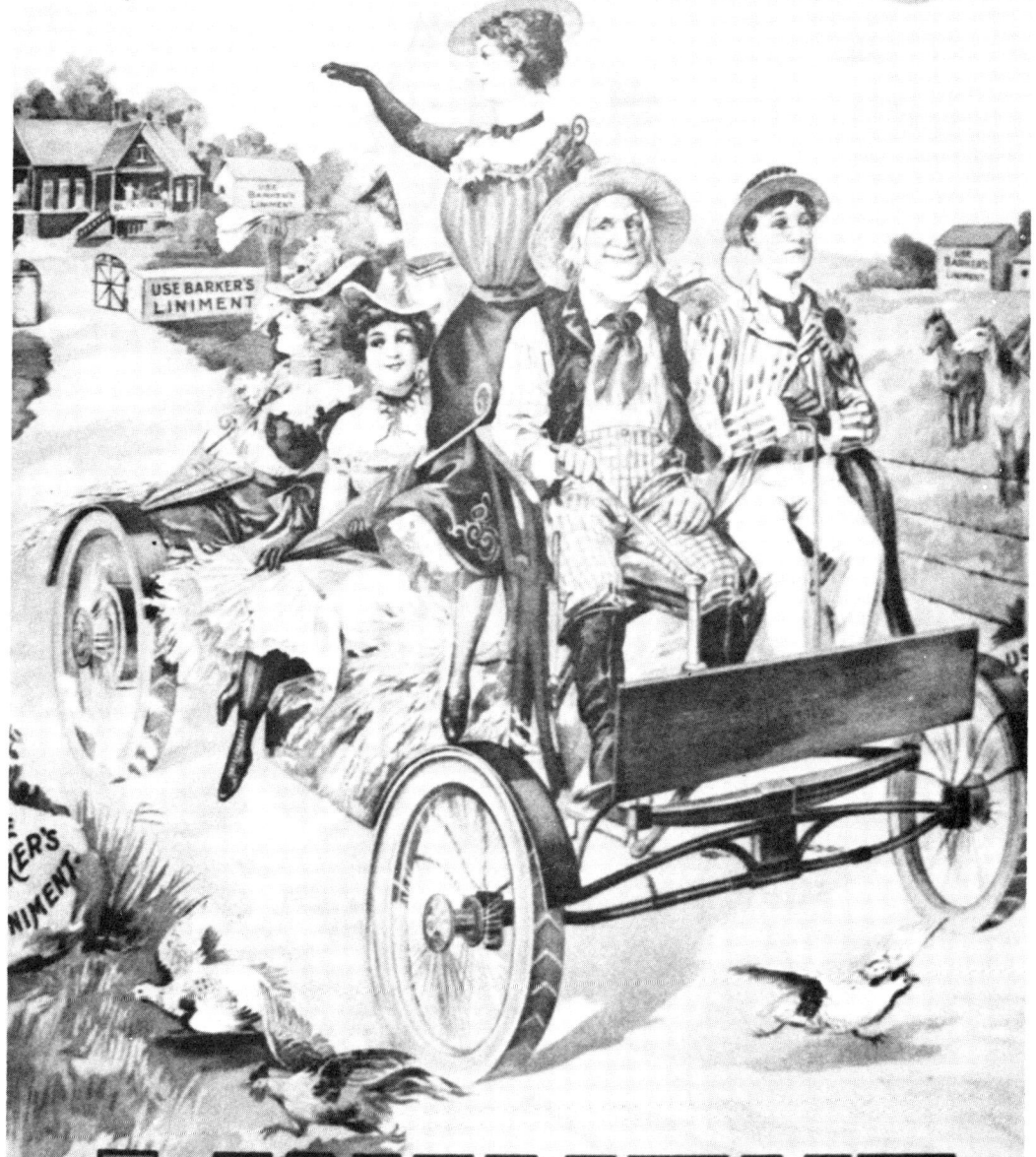

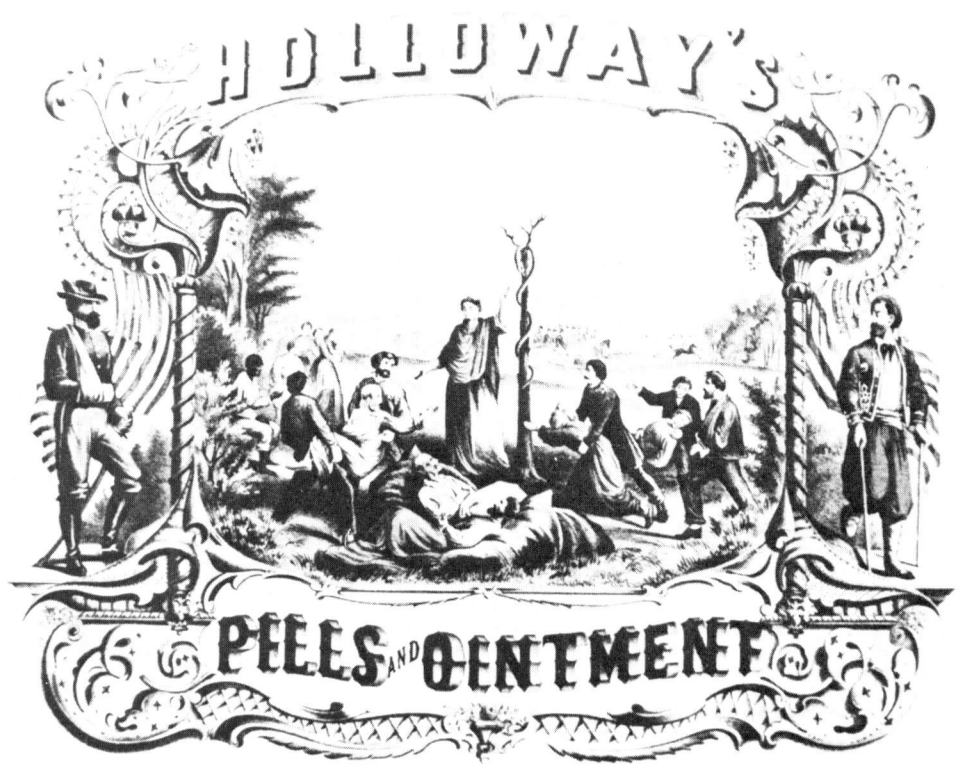
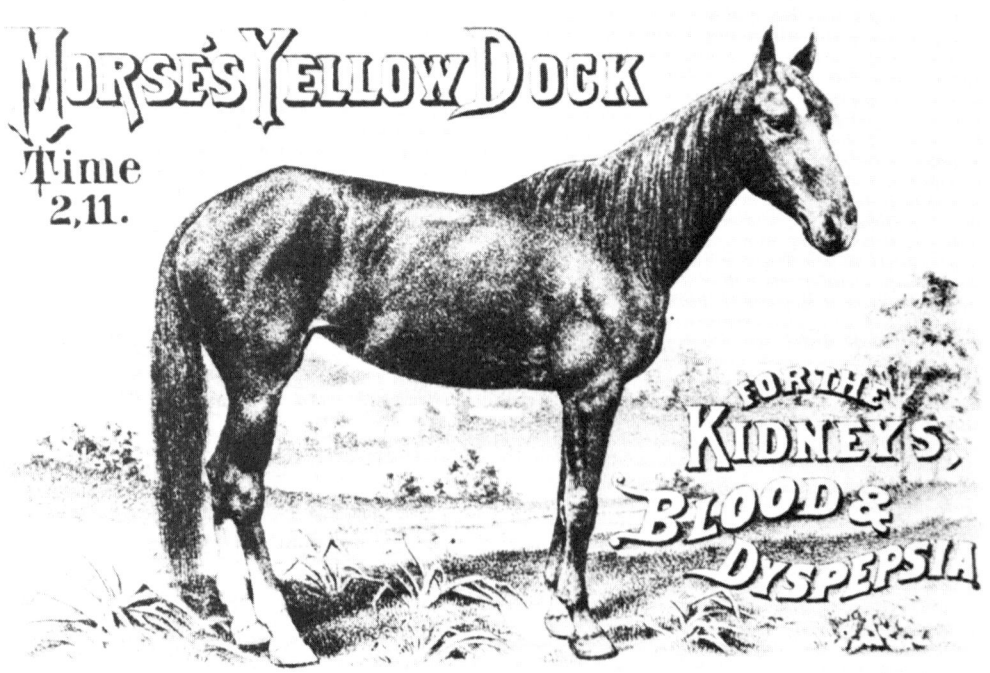

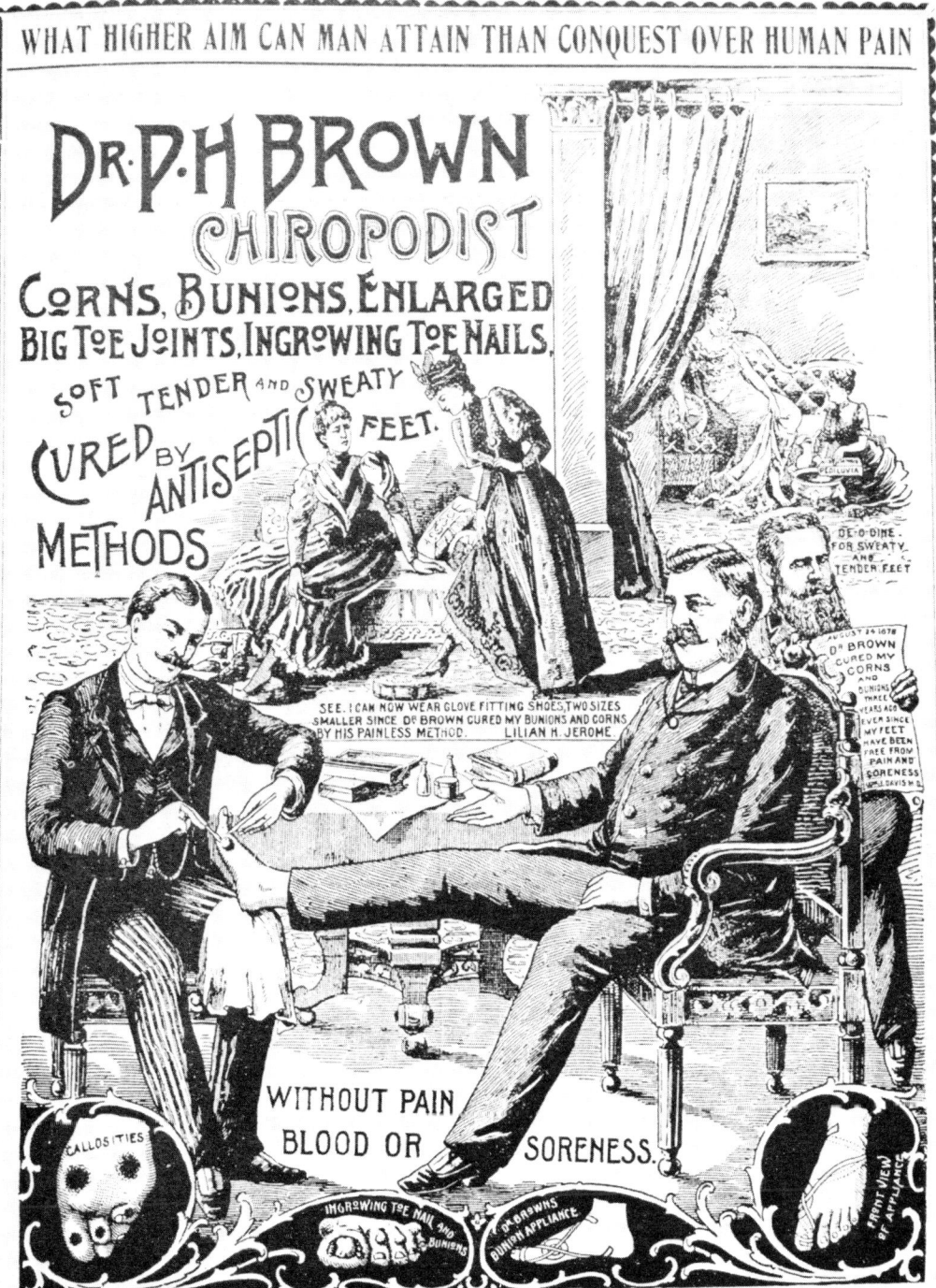

Dr Pierce's Golden Medical Discovery

The Ideal Spring Tonic and Blood Purifier

VEGETINE
The Great Blood Purifier

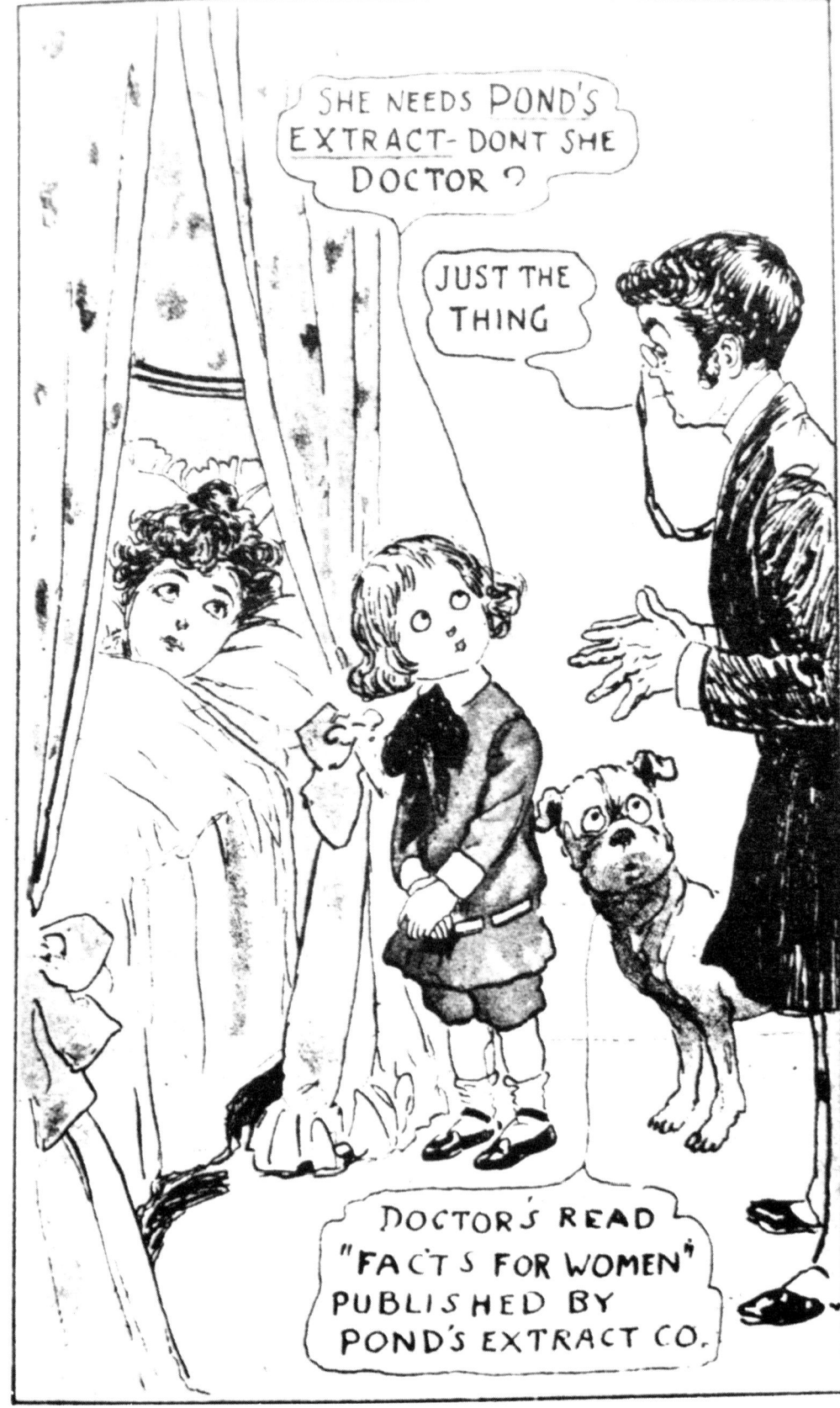

USE THE PARR ENGLISH PAD,

ABSOLUTELY HARMLESS
PERFECTLY RELIABLE

SAFE & EFFECTUAL AT ANY AND ALL TIMES.

A CERTAIN CURE FOR ALL MALARIAL OR CONTAGIOUS DISEASES

WITHOUT DRUGGING THE SYSTEM

FOR SALE BY

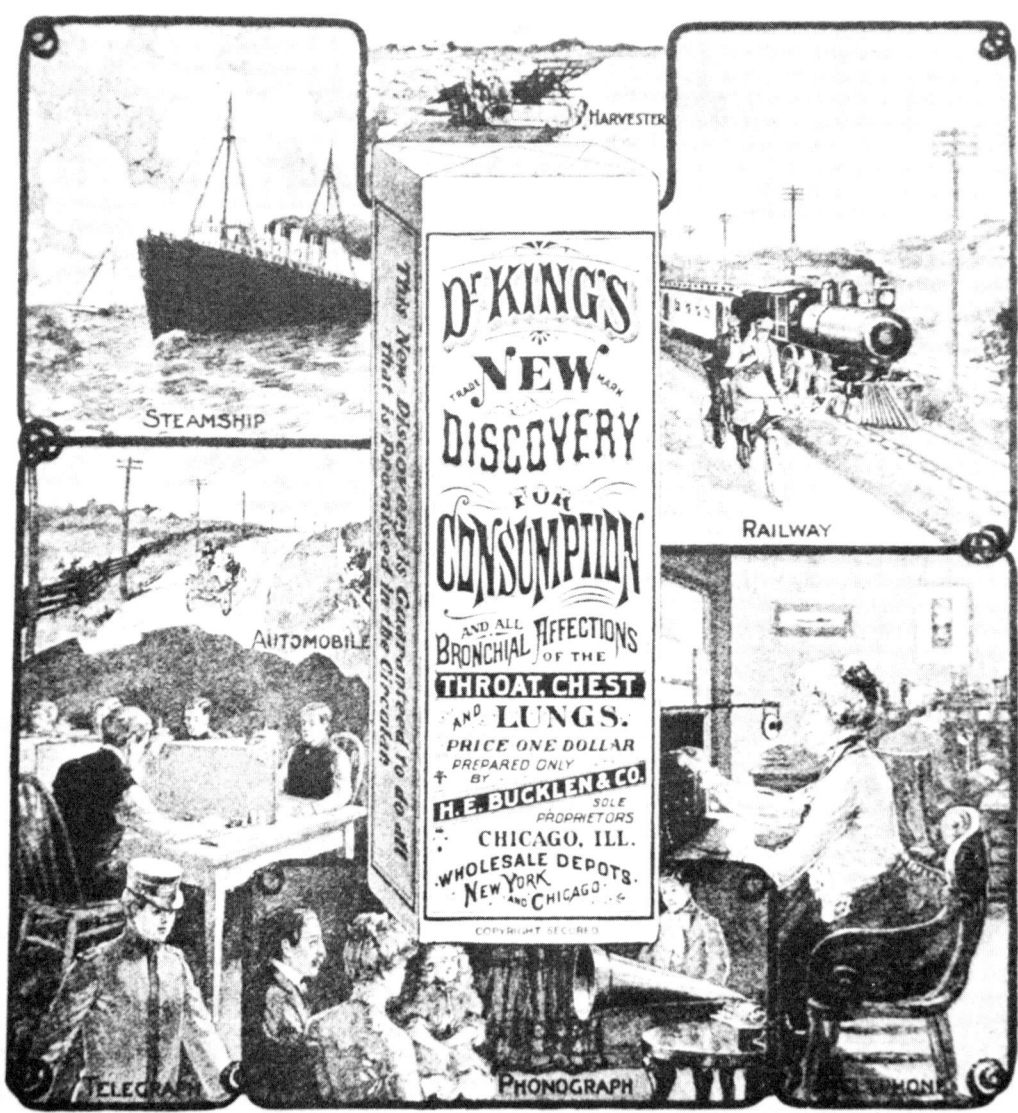

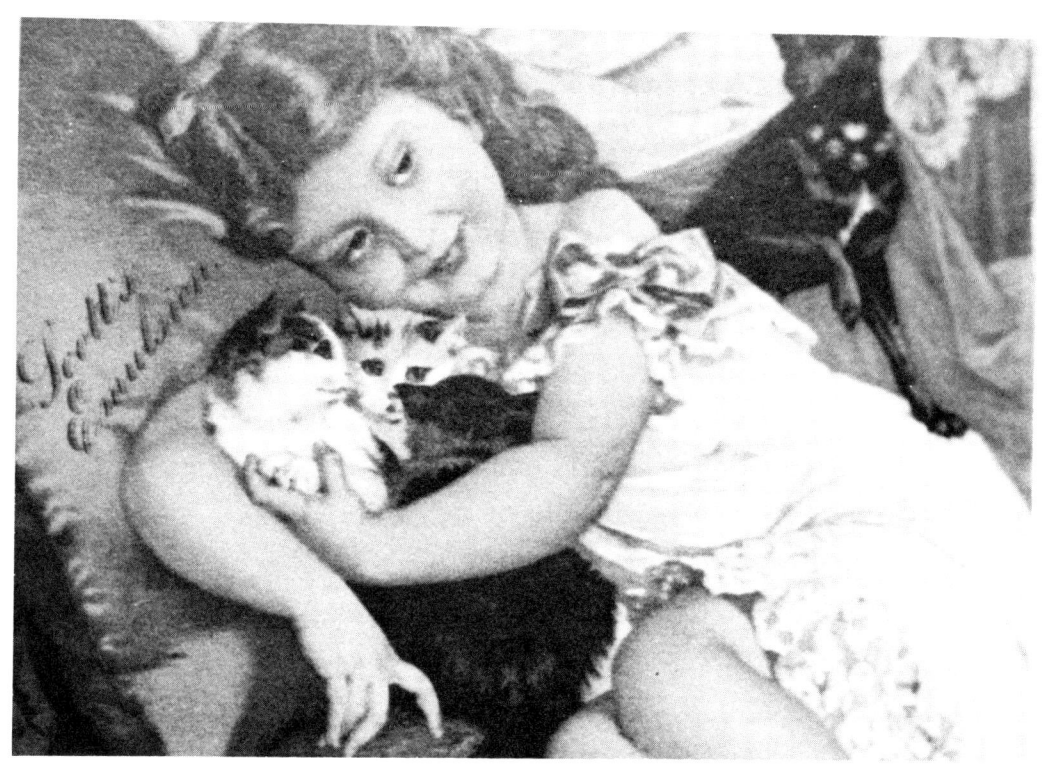

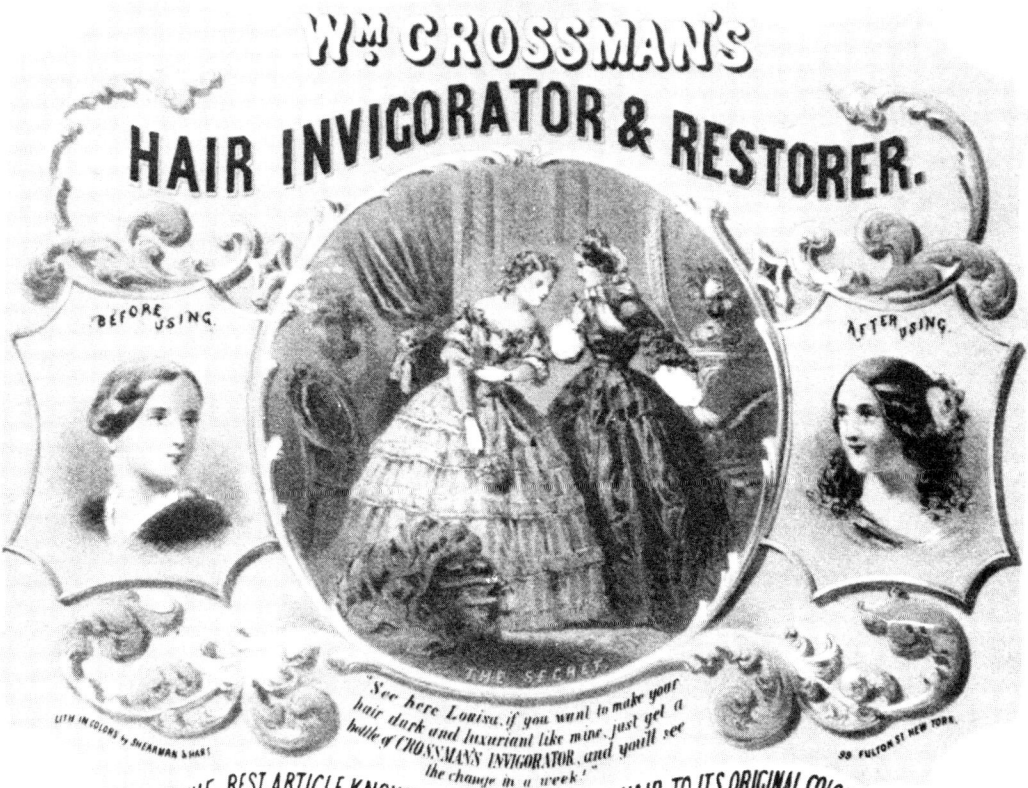

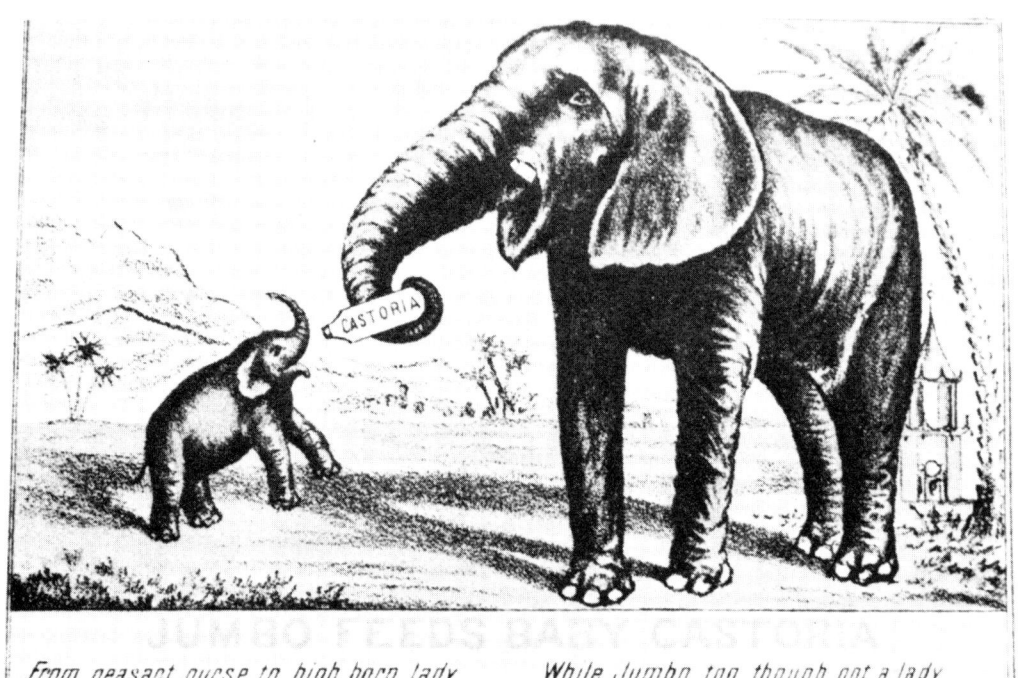

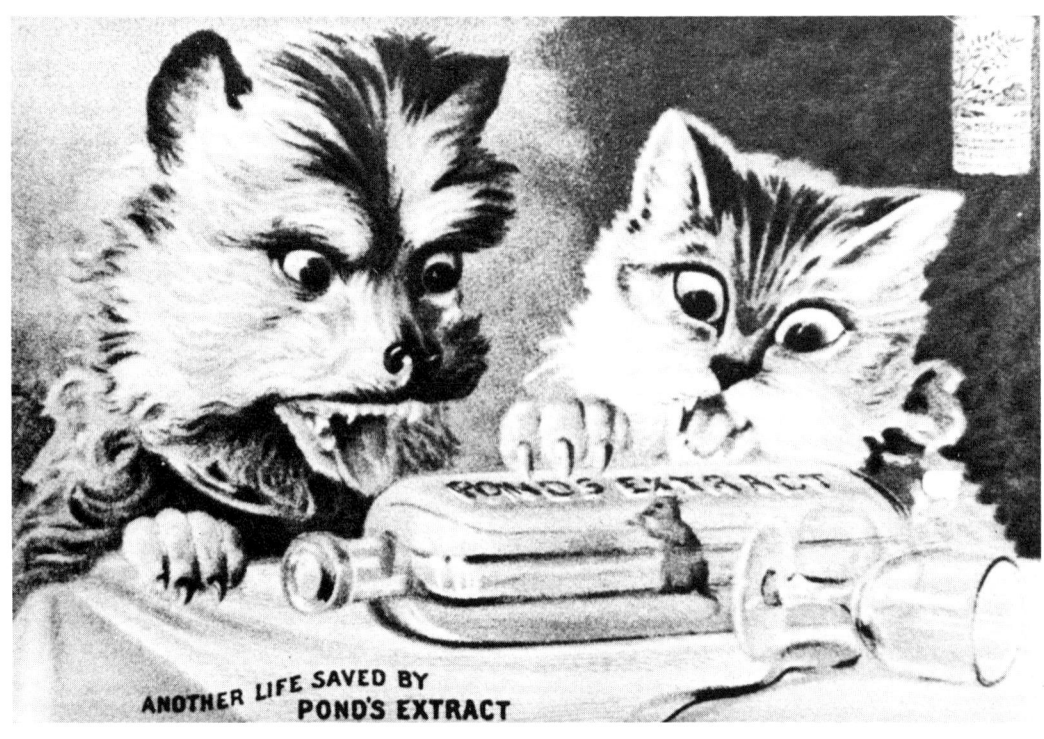

"OUR TRUST"

VEGETINE

THE GREAT BLOOD PURIFIER.

Vegetable
KEMP'S
Pastilles
for expelling
WORMS
from the System

MRS WINSLOWS
SOOTHING
SYRUP
FOR CHILDREN TEETHING

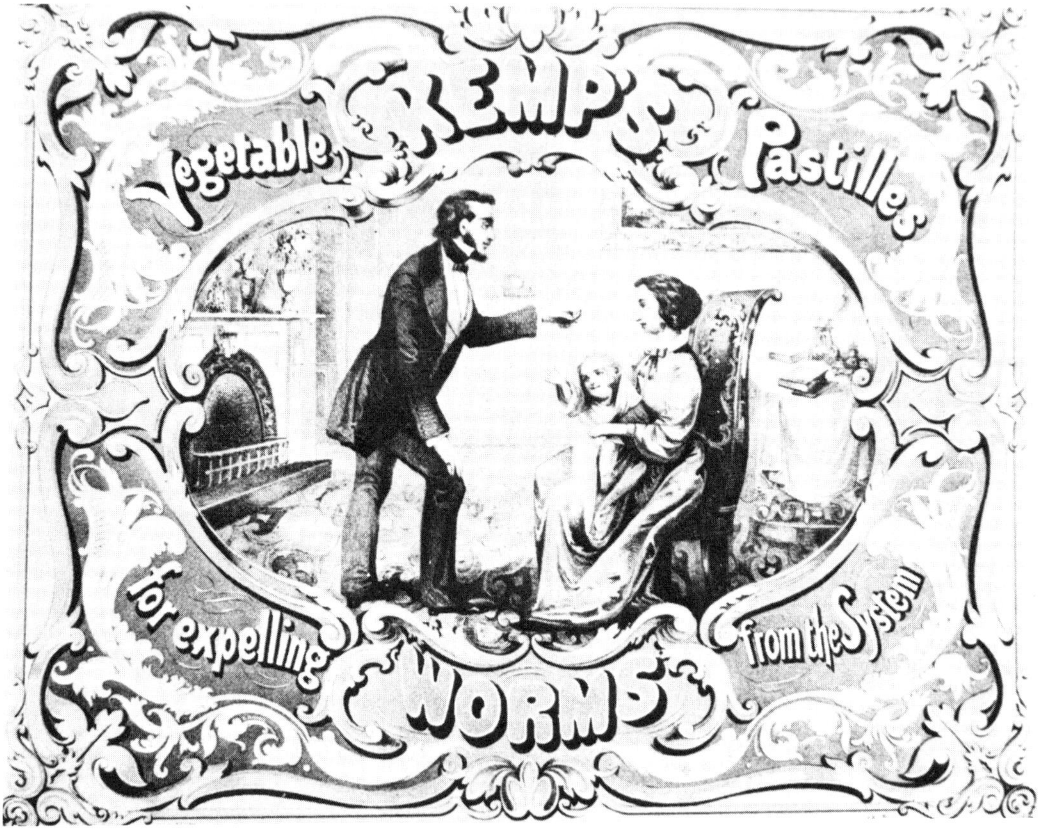

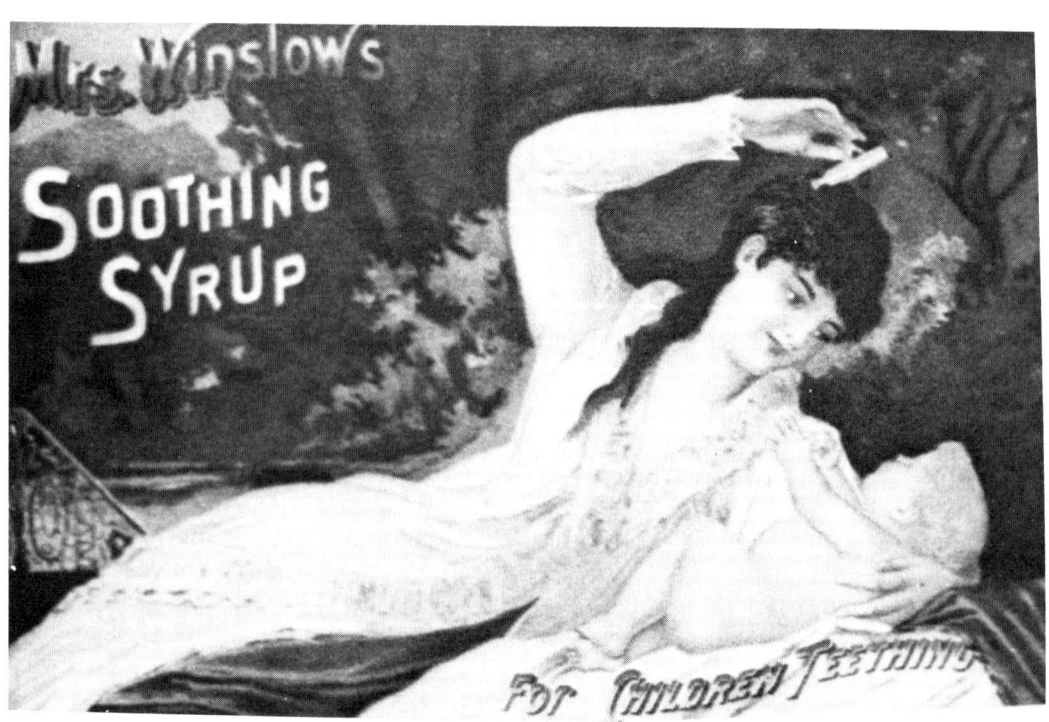

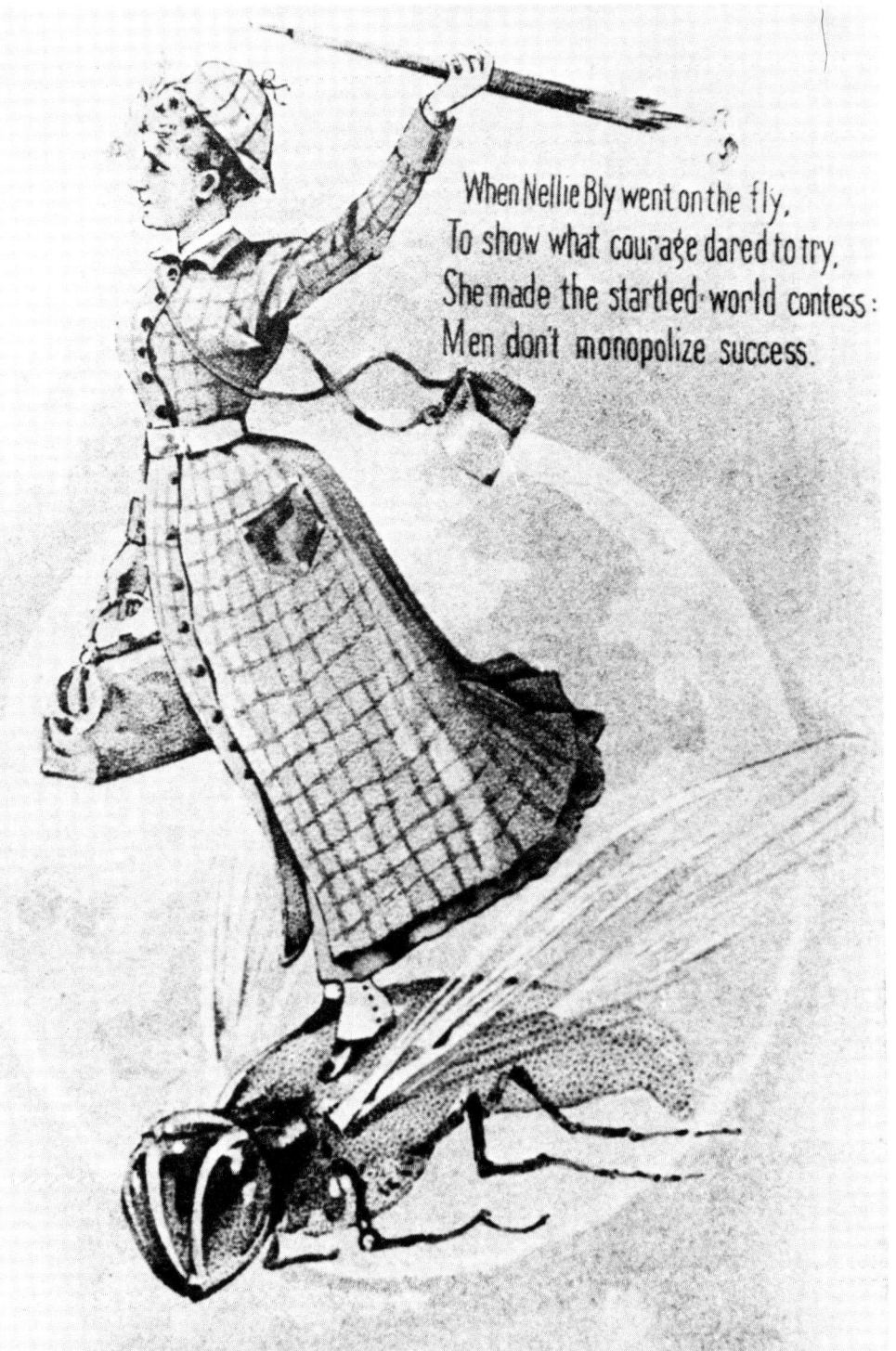

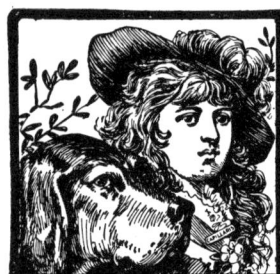
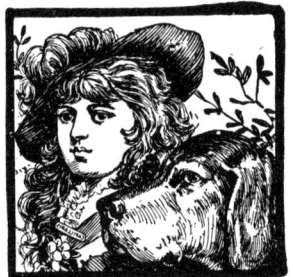

The SUPREME CURATIVE POWER of T. HILL MANSFIELD'S Capillaris

Sold by all Druggists in the U. S., or by Mail, 50c. bottle.

Has created an unprecedented sale throughout the United States without advertising. Hundreds of thousands of sufferers from all forms of skin diseases have been triumphantly cured after being given up as hopeless by physicians, hospitals and celebrated professors of medical colleges.

Quickly **Cures** sunburn, all insects, coughing, sore throat, croup, baby humors, piles, burns, cuts, poison (oak or ivy). Stings and bites of including tarantulas and centipedes, are neutralized by this scientific compound.

This remarkable remedy absolutely controls and positively cures not only the serious diseases of the **Skin** and mucuous membranes, but it is also the one hair dressing that keeps the scalp clean, white and cool — in that perfect state of health which insures an abundance of soft, luxurious hair.

CAPILLARIS will bring rest, comfort and cure to anyone suffering with Eczema, Salt Rheum, Tetter, Erysipelas, Dandruff, Itching **Scalp,** Catarrh, Falling Hair and all Face Eruptions, the most insidious Blood Diseases, Private and Syphilitic Diseases and Tumorous Growths.

A Few of Many Physicians' Testimonials.

Mr. T. Hill Mansfield. My Dear Sir:—Knowing of great cures made by your "Capillaris," I tested its composition, finding it **entirely free** from Lead, Zinc, Sulphur, Cantharides, **or anything injurious**; have used it extensively, and concluded that the medical skill of the world, as yet, has not produced its equal for the curing of Scalp and Skin Diseases, etc. This testimonial is given for the benefit of the public and deserving proprietor. **E. C. NEAL, M. D.,** Portland, Me., Manager Deering Hospital.

The Eminent Physician, Dr. Neal, has spent a long life in hospitals in Ohio, Illinois and Maine.

Mr. T. Hill Mansfield.—I am pleased to say I have used your Capillaris with entire satisfaction in cases of **Skin Diseases and Baldness.** **AMOS M. RICH, M. D.,** Brooklyn, N. Y.

"Capillaris" is an article of superior merit. **DR. G. S. NORCROSS,** San Jose, Cal.

I have used Mansfield's Capillaris successfully, and find it **does all it is claimed to.** I recommend it to others. Very truly yours, **DR. F. THOMAS,** 118 Eddy St., San Francisco, Cal.

T. Hill Mansfield, Esq.—I have used your Capillaris in cases of **Diphtheria,** with excellent results. **It transforms the Poison** to the outside of the throat. I keep it on hand for use in my practice. Respectfully, **IRA B. CUSHING, M. D.,** Brooklyn, N. Y.

A Wonderful Production, a great Public Benefit. I use it and recommend it. Use my name all you please in its behalf. **B. B. FOSTER, M. D.,** Portland, Me.

I have used Capillaris for the worst scalp disease and dandruff I ever knew of, which defied the best medical skill. It cured me, also another member of my family. These facts ought to be known to the public. **REV. F. SOUTHWORTH,** Portland, Me.

Having used T. Hill Mansfield's "Capillaris" personally and as a family medicine, I find it **an article of genuine merit,** and consider any person a public benefactor who places so valuable an article **at the disposal of an intelligent public at so low a price;** therefore it gives me pleasure to recommend it. **REV. J. L. CAMPBELL,** Madison Street Baptist Church, New York City.

Having used "Capillaris" in my practice, seen the effects of its use extensively in **severe cases of** Skin and Scalp Diseases, Catarrh, Colds, etc., etc., I can testify to its great value. **DR. JAMES CARTER,** Georgetown, Mo.

People in Alkaline and Tropical Climates! "Capillaris" will **positively** keep your head clean, cool, free from dandruff and itching.

Address T. Hill Mansfield, Agent, Glen Ridge, N. J.

DR FLINT'S
QUAKER BITTERS
DR FLINT'S QUAKER BITTERS
I take Quaker Bitters.
Quaker Bitters will restore thy health.
So will I in future.
PROVIDENCE
PREPARED BY
DR. H. S. FLINT & Co.
FOR SALE HERE

WILLIAMS'
NEW ENGLAND
COUGH REMEDY
ONE DOZ.
WILLIAMS' COUGH REMEDY
THE GREAT
FAMILY MEDICINE
FOR
COUGHS, COLDS &c.
WILLIAMS & CARLETON, PROPRIETORS.
HARTFORD, CONN.

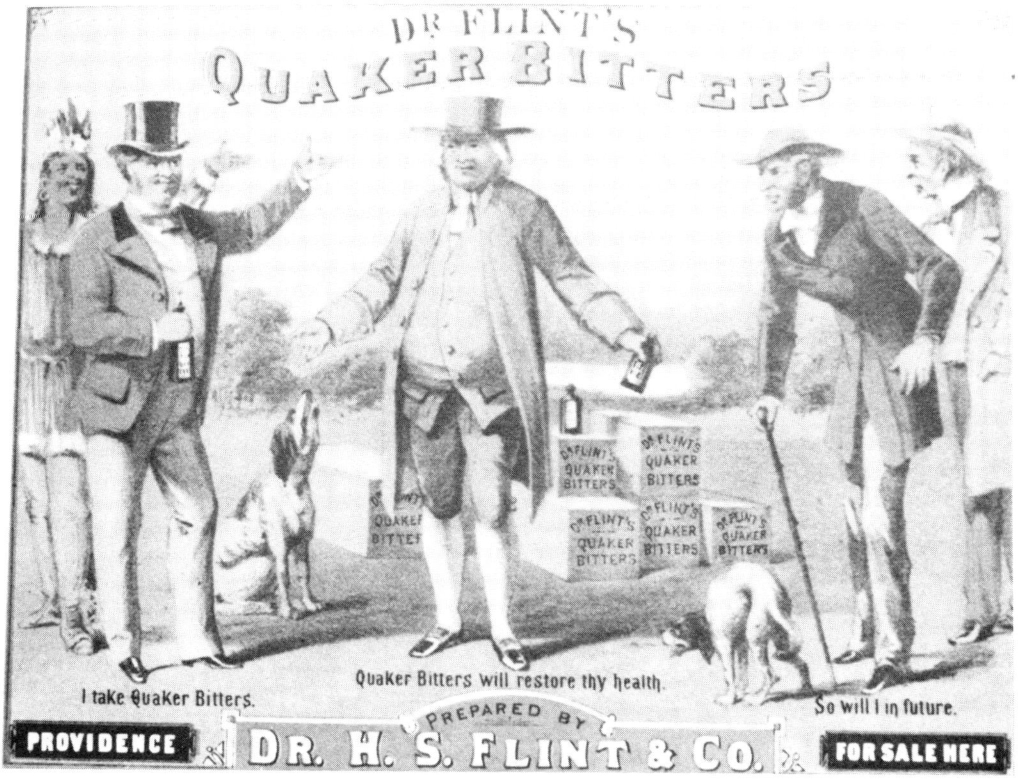

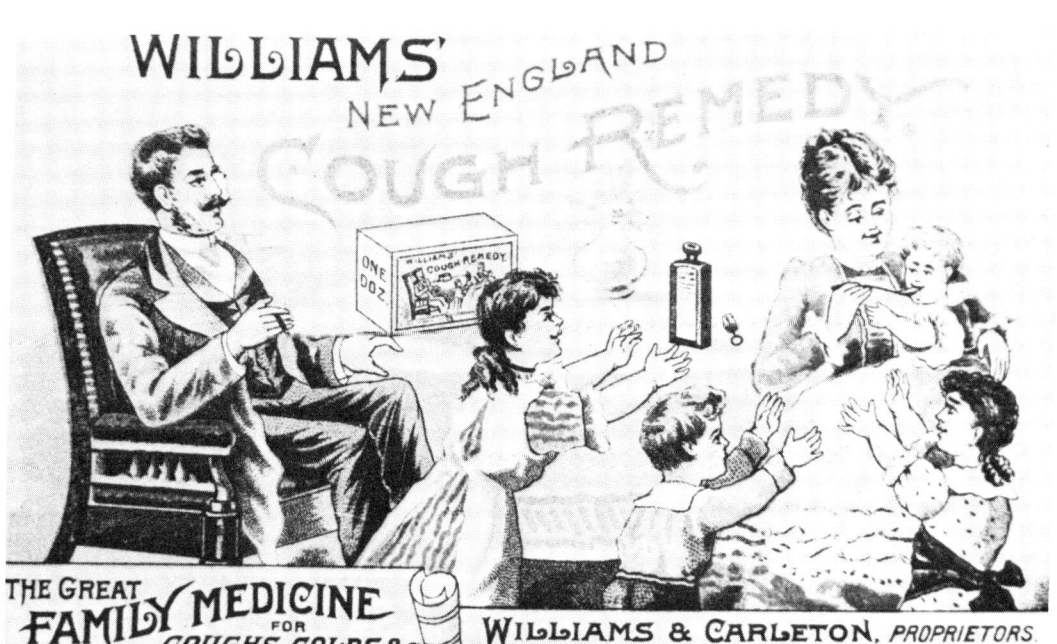

As rust and decay rapidly consume the machine that is not kept in use, so disease and sickness accumulate on the frame of indolence, until existence becomes a burden, and the grave a bed of rest.
(*The Mother's Book Of Daily Duties,* 1855)

It is well to have those who attend upon young children habituated to pleasant tones, and clear, distinct pronunciation and accent. I have seen children whose indistinct utterance and awkward manner of speaking could be traced to individuals with whom they had early intercourse. The parent must remember that every organ, every sense, every feeling, is subject to improvement, and is influenced by its early education.
(*New England Almanack,* 1840)

Beverages

"A Kind of Drink Called Rum"

It's no wonder the colonials consumed so much alcohol. Just read this 18th century description of well-water: "...well-water is most fit for consumption, however, the chief substances found in most water are pure, inflammable, and hepatic airs; acid of chalk, the fixed alkalies, vitriolated, muriated, cretised; the vegetable, oftener intrated; cretised volatile alkalies; muriated barytes; lime, and sometimes magnesia, vitriolated, nitrated, and subcretised; sometimes clay, super-vitriolated and muriated; iron, vitriolated, muriated, cretised; manganese, muriated; copper, vitriolated; calx of arsenic; petroleum; vegetable and animal putrescent mucilage...."

Another influencing factor was that most of the business of daily social and political life was conducted at the local tavern. All through the chronicles of Early America we find Washington, Henry, Jefferson, Revere, and their peers meeting in various taverns. Some of these taverns are still in existence; perhaps the most famous are Bump's Tavern in Cooperstown,

New York, and Fraunce's Tavern in lower Manhattan.

Town meetings, military musters, barn-raising parties, the posting of public notices—even executions took place at the tavern. Right up until the late 1800s hangings were considered a most important social event and great droves of the local citizenry turned out for an afternoon of drinking and gore!

The local general store encouraged drinking, too. Next to the barrel of "Black Strap" (rum mixed with molasses) was the inspiration for the bowl of peanuts at your local bar. A salted codfish hung near the barrel and the customer would occasionally reach over and grab a strip of fish, which would immediately make him buy another drink of black strap to quench the thirst created by the oversalted cod!

By 1686 the consumption of rum was so great that Increase Mather wrote, "It is an unhappy thing that in later years a Kind of Drink called Rum has been common among us. They that are poor, and wicked too, can for a penny or two-pence make themselves drunk."

But the majority of the population was vehemently pro-alcohol. In the late 1700s it was a strongly held opinion that liquor was necessary to maintain the morale of laborers, particularly farm workers. Indeed, drink was considered such a necessity that the citizens of Pennsylvania rose up in arms when the government placed an excise tax on whiskey. On August 7, 1794, President Washington had to call out the militia to put down the uprising there, which later became known as the "Whiskey Rebellion."

An excellent illustration of how attitudes concerning alcohol differed is taken from the writings of Charles Francis Adams on the habits of his relative, John Adams, the second president of the United States. "... to the end of his life a large tankard of hard cider was his morning draught before breakfast." (To put this into modern terms it would be comparable to starting out your day with a can or two of malt liquor.) Things certainly have changed—then it was *acceptable* for the president to start his day off with a quick drink!

Rather than leave you with the impression that John Adams was irresponsible, let me quote from his journal. "... if the ancients drank wine as our people drink rum it is no wonder we hear of so many possessed with devils...."

Since most of these receipts are for beverages you've never heard of, here are a few quick definitions (see the glossary if there are any others that aren't familiar):

CORDIAL: an aromatized and sweetened spirit; a liqueur.
CREAM: a syrupy liqueur.
LIQUEUR: a spiritous liquor flavored with an aromatic substance.
POSSET: a beverage of hot milk, curdled by ale, wine, etc. and spiced.
PUNCH: a beverage usually composed of wine or distilled liquor, water, milk, or tea, with sugar, lemon juice, and often mint or spice.
RATAFIA: any liquor flavored with fruit and/or fruit kernels.

"Good rum properly diluted with water, sweetened with sugar, and drunk with moderation, strengthens the lax fibres, incrassates the thin fluids, and warms the habit. It proves most beneficial to those exposed to heat, moisture, corrupted air, and putrid diseases."

(*Stearns' Herbal,* 1801)

Possets, Cordials & Punches

What better way to start out than with a...
BANG: Take a pint of cider, and add to a pint of warm ale; sweeten with treacle or sugar to taste, grate in some nutmeg and ginger, and add a wineglassful of gin or whiskey.

(*Practical Housewife,* 1860)

This is a nice, light, summer drink. If you use blackcurrant syrup for the sweetening and garnish it with a fresh mint leaf, you'll end up with one of the nicest substitutes for that everyday pitcher of lemonade.
SHERRY COBBLER: Take some very fine and clean ice, break into small pieces, fill a tumbler to within an inch of the top with it, put a table-spoonful of plain syrup, capillaire, or any other flavor—some prefer strawberry—add the quarter of the zest of a lemon, and add a few drops of the juice. Fill with sherry, stir it up, and let it stand five or six minutes. Sip it gently through a straw.

(*Practical Housewife,* 1860)

This receipt has always struck me as the creation of some 18th century alcoholic healthfood addict....

OXFORD NIGHTCAP: Take half a tumbler of tea, made as usual with sugar and milk, add a slice of lemon, a wine-glass of new milk, and the same of rum or brandy; beat up a new-laid egg, and add to the whole while warm.

(*Practical Housewife,* 1860)

Here's a nice posset to serve after skating or shoveling snow off the driveway. "Crumb of a penny loaf grated fine" means breadcrumbs made from the remains of a loaf of bread the colonials referred to as a "penny loaf"—the modern equivalent would be the crumbs made from one slice of white bread.

ORANGE POSSET: Take the crumb of a penny loaf grated fine, and put into half a pint of water, with half the peel of a Seville orange grated, or sugar which has been rubbed upon the peel. Boil all together, till it looks thick and clear; then take the juice of half a Seville orange, beat well with a tablespoonful of brandy, add sugar to taste, and a pint of white or raisin wine; mix well, add to the posset, and serve.

(old manuscript cookery book)

Lemon posset is a very substantial drink; we have nothing today that resembles it, except perhaps lemon yoghurt. This was considered a very elegant drink to be served at weddings and important functions. It's very interesting to try but I suggest you halve the receipt so you'll end up with a usable amount. And please remember to whisk in *one* direction only, otherwise you'll end up with a mess that looks like cottage cheese!

LEMON POSSET: Steep the rind of a lemon pared thin, in a pint of sweet white wine two hours before required, add the juice of one lemon, add sugar to taste; put it in a bowl with a quart of milk or cream, and whisk one way till very thick. This will fill twenty glasses, which may be filled the day before required.

(*Practical Housewife,* 1860)

Royal posset is a sort of glorified, very rich eggnog. Though the ale of colonial times was much more like Guinness stout than our Ballantine ale, today's palates are likely to prefer the mildness of contemporary ale in this receipt. Please don't let it come to a boil or you'll end up with a very unpalatable, scalded failure.

ROYAL POSSET: Take half a pint of ale, mix a pint of cream with it; then add the yolks of four eggs and the whites of two well beaten, sweeten to taste and flavour with nutmeg. Pour into a saucepan, set it over the fire, stir well until thick, and before it boils, remove; pour into a basin and serve hot.

(*Practical Housewife,* 1860)

Recently I saw an ad for strawberry cordial—"Finally we've been able to capture the real flavor of strawberries in a delicious liqueur..." The small print said "artificially flavored." Well, here's a receipt for strawberry cordial that's been around for at least a hundred and fifty years and it's naturally flavored!

STRAWBERRY CORDIAL: Hull a sufficient quantity of ripe strawberries, and squeeze them through a linen bag. To each quart of the juice allow a pint of white brandy, and half a pound of powdered loaf sugar. Put the liquid into a glass jar or demijohn, and let it stand a fortnight. Then filter through a sieve, to the bottom of which a fine piece of muslin has been fastened; and afterwards bottle it.

(*Miss Leslie's Complete Cookery,* 1839)

Raspberry cordial is a really delicious after-dinner drink and very easy to make. If you live in an area where raspberries are to be had for the picking in the early summer, it's a must! I like it so much I make it even when I have to buy the raspberries. I prefer to use 100-proof vodka in place of the whiskey as more of the fruit flavor comes through.

RASPBERRY CORDIAL: To each quart of raspberries allow a pound of loaf-sugar. Mash the raspberries and strew the sugar over them, having first pounded it slightly, or cracked it with a rolling-pin. Let the raspberries and sugar set till the next day, keeping them well-covered, then put them in a thin linen bag and squeeze out all the juice with your hands. To every pint of juice allow a quart of double-rectified whiskey. Cork it well, and set it away for use. It will be ready in a few days.

(*Seventy-five Receipts,* 1838)

Here's a receipt for a cordial that is simply unavailable commercially. A small glass of this in the middle of the winter will make all the work it took to make it seem trifling. Oh, and a little of this poured over vanilla ice cream is sublime!

PEACH CORDIAL: Take a peck of cling-stone peaches; such as come late in the season, and are very juicy. Pare them, and cut them from the stones. Crack about half the stones and save the kernels. Leave the remainder of the stones whole, and mix them with the cut peaches; also add the kernels. Put the whole into a wide-mouthed demi-john, and pour on them two gallons of double-rectified whiskey. Add three pounds of rock-sugar candy. Cork it tightly, and set away for three months; then bottle it, and it will be fit for use. It will be improved in clearness by covering the bottom of a sieve with blotting paper (secured with pins) and straining the cordial through it.

(Seventy-five Receipts, 1838)

Just the name of this drink is reason enough to include it...

PERFECT LOVE: Zests of lemon, two ounces; zests of lime, four ounces; cloves, two drachms; alcohol, two and a half gallons; sugar, ten pounds; water, two quarts. Macerate ten days in the alcohol, then filtrate and bottle.

(The Art of Confectionery, 1866)

Vinegar has long been considered very healthful in conjunction with honey, so in this receipt replace the sugar with honey and you'll have a super-healthful Raspberry Shrub—a real thirst quencher on a hot summer afternoon.

RASPBERRY SHRUB: Raspberry shrub mixed with water is a pure, delicious drink for summer; and in a country where raspberries are abundant, it is good economy to make it answer instead of Port or Catalonia wine. Put raspberries in a pan, and scarcely cover them with strong vinegar. Add a pint of sugar to a pint of the juice; (of this you can judge by first trying your pan to see how much it will hold); scald it, skim it, and bottle it when cold. Upon drinking you may add brandy or rum.

(American Frugal Housewife, 1833)

Shrubs can be mixed with club soda, water, wine, vodka—just about anything you'd like. This particular receipt contains rum, but you can use any other alcohol. Vodka is also very good in this one.

CURRANTSHRUB: Strip the fruit, and prepare in a jar as for jelly; strain the juice, of which put two quarts to one gallon of rum, and two pounds of lump sugar; strain through a jelly-bag and bottle.

(Domestic Cookery, 1807)

This is great to have in your pantry—just mix with water or club soda for a very sophisticated lemonade.

LEMON SHRUB: Pare a thin rind off from fresh lemons; squeeze out and strain the juice; put to a pint of it, a pound of sugar broken into small pieces; take for each pint of the syrup three spoonfuls of brandy, and soak the rind of the lemon in it. Let all stand one day, frequently stirring up the lemon juice and sugar. Next day pour off the syrup, and mix with it the brandy and lemon rinds. Keep it all under sealed corks, in dry sand, in a cool place.

(*Book of Receipts,* 1858)

Liquodilla is another variation of the lemon & orange & brandy beverages, but I couldn't resist including it because I like the name so much!

LIQUODILLA: Take the thin peel of 6 oranges and 6 lemons, steep them in a gallon of brandy or rum, close stopped, for 2 or 3 days; then take 6 quarts of water, and 3 pounds of loaf sugar. Let it boil a quarter of an hour, then strain it through a fine sieve, and let it stand until cold; strain the brandy from the peels, and add the juice of 5 oranges and 7 lemons to each gallon. Keep it close stopped up for 6 weeks, then bottle it.

(*Mackenzie's 5000 Receipts,* 1829)

The fine line between medicinal beverages and just plain serious drinking is a nebulous one at best, but this cordial was usually drunk for pleasure rather than illness.

CHERRY CORDIAL: Take Black Cherries, large and full ripe, plucking off their stalks only, 12 pounds, put them in a large Stone Bottle, to which put choice brandy six Quarts, Double Refined Loaf Sugar, 3 pounds in Powder, Lime Juice a pint and a half, Cinnamon bruised, Cloves slit, Nutmegs bruised, of each a quarter of an Ounce; stop them up close, shaking the Bottle once every day; After three weeks you may use it; Two, Three, or Four Spoonfuls, will be an extraordinary Cordial, at any time upon Fainting, or Illness, especially in a morning Fasting.

(*Dr. Salmon's Recipes,* 1710)

This is much nicer than commercial creme de menthe since it isn't as sweet or artificially colored. You needn't add the water, and why not experiment a bit—one year I made this with bourbon in place of the brandy and got sort of an instant Mint Julep.

MINT CORDIAL: Pick the mint early in the morning while the dew is on it, and be careful not to bruise it; pour some water over it and drain it—put two handsful into a pitcher, with a quart of French brandy, cover it, and let it stand till the next day; take the mint carefully out, and put in as much more, which must be taken out the next day—do this the third time; then put three quarts of water to the brandy, and one pound of loaf sugar powdered; mix it well together—and when perfectly clear, bottle it.

(*Virginia Housewife,* 1856)

This is probably the most famous of the colonial drinks, and still a great favorite wherever people must endure cold winters. (The term "Rum-Grog" means rum diluted with boiling water.)

BUTTERED TODDY: Mix a glass of rum-grog pretty strong and hot, sweeten to taste with honey, flavour with nutmeg and lemon-juice, and add a piece of fresh butter the size of a walnut.

(*Practical Housewife*, 1860)

This is a very basic punch, quite similar to many of the punches we make today. I suggest substituting club soda or ginger ale for the water, and the "wine-glassful of maraschino" is easily replaced with half a jar of maraschino cherries with their juice.

PUNCH, COLD: Pour half a pint of gin on the rind of a lemon; add a table-spoonful of lemon juice, a wine-glassful of maraschino, a pint and a half of water, and two bottles of iced water.

(*Practical Housewife*, 1860)

This punch is easy to make, delicious, and a real treat for those occasions when you want something special and out of the ordinary. You needn't add the tea, though I suggest replacing the water with champagne. Use an inexpensive domestic brand and you'll be rewarded with a very special punch.

PUNCH A LA ROMAINE: Take a quart of lemon ice, add the whites of three eggs well beaten, with rum and brandy, till the ice liquifies, in the proportion of three parts of rum to one of brandy, and water to taste. Then add a teacupful of strong green tea infusion, strained, and a little champagne.

(*Practical Housewife*, 1860)

If you're a Southern Comfort drinker this receipt will become one of your favorites. Just replace the whiskey with Southern Comfort and omit the sugar.

SCOTCH PUNCH, OR WHISKEY TODDY (The Duke Of Athol's Receipt): Pour about a wine-glassful of boiling water into a half-pint tumbler, and add sugar according to taste. Stir well up, then mix a wine-glassful of whiskey, and add a wine-glassful and a half more boiling water. *Be sure the water is boiling!* Never put lemon

Epitaph on a Hard Drinker: Old Bibo would tipple to moisten his clay;
And Tippled so much that he washed it away.
(*Farmer's Almanack*, 1799)

into toddy. The two in combination, in almost every instance, produce acidity upon the stomach. If possible, store your whiskey in the wood, not in bottles, as the keeping in the barrel mellows it, and takes away the coarser particles.

(*Practical Housewife,* 1860)

I haven't the slightest idea why these drinks were named in honor of bishops and cardinals, but they've always been among my favorite colonial receipts because their names intrigue me. Oh, and please disregard the instructions to use an old bottle of wine—a domestic jug variety is just fine for a punch.

BISHOP: Take three smooth-skinned and large Seville oranges, and grill them to a pale brown colour over a clear, slow fire; then place in a small punchbowl that will about hold them, and pour over them half a pint from a bottle of old Bordeaux wine, in which a pound and a quarter of loaf sugar is dissolved; then cover with a plate, and let stand for two days. When it is to be served, cut and squeeze the oranges into a small sieve above a jug containing the remainder of the bottle of sweetened Bordeaux, previously made very hot, and if when mixed it is not sweet enough, add more sugar. Serve hot in tumblers. Some persons make Bishop with raisin or Lisbon wine, and add mace or cloves or nutmegs, but this is not the proper way.

CARDINAL: Is made the same way as Bishop, substituting old Rhenish wine for the Bordeaux.

(*Practical Housewife,* 1860)

And now the receipt for the original "Boiler Maker"!

COOL TANKARD: Put into a quart of mild ale a wine-glassful of white wine, the same of brandy and capillaire, the juice of a lemon, and a little piece of the rind. Add a sprig of borage or balm, a bit of toasted bread and nutmeg grated on the top.

(*Practical Housewife,* 1860)

Liquors

The colonials flavored their alcohol with infinite imagination, often with substances we're not familiar with. No longer do we flavor with such ingredients as jasmine blossoms, pomegranates or apricot kernels, which is why these receipts are so much fun to make. Re-creating flavors and aromas that were commonplace two hundred years ago is a very rewarding and interesting experience. But be careful—you just might end up a fanatic like me!

Why not make up several different types and then bottle them up in small medicine bottles (available at your drugstore), then give them as gifts this holiday season. I've found just about everyone loves to receive this as an extra-special present, and it's just perfect for those people-who-have-everything. I can almost guarantee even the best-stocked liquor cabinet doesn't contain Raspberry Ratafia!

Here's another rose-flavored receipt—this time for brandy. The process is very simple and you can vary the proportions to make as much or as little as you like; your only limitation is how many rose petals you can get your hands on. I have a helpful neighbor with a large rose garden, but for those of you who aren't as fortunate, you can always substitute oil or essence of roses and get good results.

> ROSE BRANDY: Gather petals from fragrant roses without bruising, fill a pitcher with them, and cover them with French brandy; next day, pour off the brandy, take out the petals, and fill the pitcher with fresh ones, and return the brandy; do this until it is strongly impregnated, then bottle it up; keep the pitcher closely covered during the process. It is better than distilled rose water for cakes &c.

(Virginia Housewife, 1856)

If you're like me and prefer your brandy fruitier than those commercially available, this receipt is just what you've been looking for. If you can't get fresh raspberries I've found you can use raspberry syrup with very excellent results—just remember to cut down on the amount of sugar because the raspberry syrup is already sweetened.

> RASPBERRY BRANDY: Pick fine, dry fruit, put into a stone jar, and the jar into a kettle of water, or on a hot hearth, till the juice will run; strain, and to every pint add half a pound of sugar, give one boil, and skim it; when cold, put equal quantities of juice and brandy, shake well, and bottle. Some people prefer it stronger of the brandy.

(Domestic Cookery, 1807)

A gentleman in Virginia, writes to a friend in Richmond for a still of certain dimensions and thus expresses himself:—"Sir, I want a Still maid that will work thirty-six gallants." [He meant gallons].

(Allan's New England Almanack, 1811)

Jasmine Cream is delicious, exotic, and, if you use commercial orange-flower water and tincture of jasmine, very easy to make.

>JASMINE CREAM: Dissolve over the fire two pounds of double-refined sugar in a quart of water; let it cool, and add three ounces of double-distilled tincture of jasmine, four drachms of orange-flower water, and one and a half pints of alcohol; mix the whole well, filter, and bottle for use.
>
>Sugar, 2 lbs.; water, 1 qt.; jasmine, 3 oz.; orange-flower water, 4 drs.; alcohol, 1½ pts.

(The Art Of Confectionery, 1866)

This receipt yields a coffee-flavored liquor which you can vary to suit your taste. Try using a French roast or espresso coffee, adding a vanilla bean, using brown sugar, molasses—the variations are almost endless and the result is your own personal blend.

>RATAFIA DE CAFE: Take of roasted coffee, ground, 1 lb.; proof spirit, 1 gallon; sugar, 20 oz. Digest for one week, then filter and bottle.

(Mackenzie's 5000 Receipts, 1829)

For those of you who live in citrus country this is a really splendid beverage. It's so pleasing to the senses that it was considered an aphrodisiac!

>RATAFIA DE FLEURS D'ORANGES: Take of fresh flowers of orange-tree, 2 lbs., proof spirit, 1 gallon,—sugar, 1½ lbs. Digest for 6 hours, filtrate, and bottle.

(Mackenzie's 5000 Receipts, 1829)

For those of us who don't happen to live near citrus groves, this receipt is the next best thing. Oh, and those miniature oranges that are grown as house plants are just perfect if you happen to have enough.

>RATAFIA D'ECORES D'ORANGES: Take of fresh peel of Seville oranges, 4 oz.—proof spirit, 1 gallon,—sugar, 1 lb. Digest for six hours, strain, and bottle.

(Mackenzie's 5000 Receipts, 1829)

From now on save your apricot and peach pits and before you know it you'll have enough to make this receipt. Keep the pits whole until it's time to use them, then crack off the shells to expose the kernels. The flavor of Ratafia de Noyeau is very similar to Amaretto.

>RATAFIA DE NOYEAU: Take of peach or apricot kernels, with their shells bruised, in number 120, proof spirit, 4 pints, sugar, 10 oz. Digest for 1 month and then strain and bottle. Some reduce the

strength of the spirit of wine with the juice of apricots or peaches to make this a liqueur.

(*Mackenzie's 5000 Receipts,* 1829)

I make this receipt using four pomegranates and one quart of brandy. The flavor is unlike anything you've ever had and I urge you to try it.

POMEGRANATE RATAFIA: Steep fifteen fully ripe pomegranates, cut in slices, in four quarts of brandy, for fifteen days; squeeze through a cloth; add a syrup made with three pounds of sugar, and filter.
Pomegranates, 15; brandy, 4 qts.; sugar, 3 lbs.; steep fifteen days.

(*The Art Of Confectionery,* 1866)

Here's another receipt that I usually cut down the proportions of: I use one pound of raspberries to a quart of brandy. If you like the raspberry flavor to be more dominant, double the amount of berries (use two pounds per quart of brandy).

RASPBERRY RATAFIA: Steep eight pounds of raspberries for fifteen days in two gallons of brandy; add a syrup made with seven pounds of sugar and filter.
Raspberries, 8 lbs.; brandy, 2 gals.; sugar, 7 lbs.; water, 3 pts. Steep fifteen days.

(*The Art Of Confectionery,* 1866)

This makes a very good drink for that bloated feeling you get after eating too much. I've never been able to determine whether the colonials used it for that purpose, but nonetheless it's the equal of the best European stomach bitters.

USQUEBAUGH: Usquebaugh is a strong compound liquor, chiefly taken by way of dram; it is made in the highest perfection at Drogheda in Ireland. The following are the ingredients, and the proportions in which they are to be used.
Take of the best brandy, 1 gallon—raisins, stoned, 1 lb.—cinnamon, cloves, nutmegs, and cardamoms, each 1 oz. crushed in a mortar,—saffron, half an ounce,—rind of one Seville orange, and brown sugar candy, 1 lb. Shake these very well every day, for at least 14 days, and it will, at the expiration of that time, be ready to be fined for use.

(*Mackenzie's 5000 Receipts,* 1829)

TEMPERANCE DRINKS

"And on they came like a torrent"

The drinking habits of the early colonists were by no means as puritanical as one might suppose, and the increased consumption of alcoholic beverages in seventeenth and eighteenth century America leaves little doubt why there was an active temperance movement beginning early in the nineteenth century.

The first national temperance group was founded on February 13, 1826. By 1833 the problem had grown to such proportions that the nation's congressmen formed the Congressional Temperance Society. Its purpose was to discourage "the use of ardent spirit and the traffick in it, by example and kind moral influence."

Records show that drinking was so widespread that by 1835 the estimated annual death toll from drink was 56,000 and "that five hundred thousand drunkards are now living in our blessed America, all moving onward to the dreadful verge. What a scene of immolation!"

This was the same year that the Cold Water Society became a major influence in the temperance movement. The Reverend Thomas P. Hunt distributed pledge cards to Sunday School students and sent them off to obtain the signatures of any nonabstainers.

The forerunner of Alcoholics Anonymous was born in 1840 with the birth of the Washington Temperance Society. The membership consisted of former heavy drinkers who gathered to tell of their experiences prior to and after taking the oath of abstinence. The society claimed to have reformed 500,000 "intemperate" drinkers and 100,000 "habitual drunkards" by 1843. One convert wrote, "A few leaders in the ranks of intemperance having signed the Pledge, it appeared to be a signal for the mass to follow; and on they came, like a torrent sweeping everything before it. It was for weeks the all-absorbing topic."

The Sons of Intemperance was established at Teetotaler's Hall in

New York City in 1842. This organization was also a fraternal society, with dues, initiation fees, and secret rituals.

Three years later another combined temperance and fraternal organization was founded in New York City—The Temple of Honor, whose membership was confined to Protestants. Although well received in the north, it was enthusiastically received in the south where they adopted a ritual involving elaborate costumes and passwords.

By 1851 there was such mounting concern over the evils of overindulgence that temperance was the favorite theme for newspaper articles, plays, and books. In 1854 one of the most successful plays was Katy, The Hot Corn Girl. *The plot involved a once-happy family brought to ruin when the father began to drink and gamble, then turned to crime to pay his debts. The wife began to imbibe, too, "the rum destroying her maternal feelings." Their poor daughter, Katy, is forced to the streets to sell hot corn to support her indigent family, catches pneumonia, and dies.*

But even amidst all this temperance propaganda there were still those who stressed the medicinal properties of alcohol.

The temperance groups realized that the alcoholic drinks had to be replaced by palatable substitutes, and they mustered all their ingenuity in creating recipes for Temperance Drinks. Many of their recipes still produce delicious beverages, and it is this era we have to thank for the invention of that modern American standby, carbonated soda.

Coffee, Ice, or Capillaire?

The following recipe from *The Farmer's Almanack*, 1815, is included here more for its entertainment value than actual use—potatoes, at least to my taste, make miserable coffee. In reading the recipe you'll probably be struck by the fact that things haven't changed as much as one might think. They were complaining about unemployment and inflation in 1815! (The recipe on "To Make Coffee" is likewise of little use to us, but it's amusing to learn how they made it in the nineteenth century.)

> POTATOE COFFEE: Frugality in domestic expenses, is a virtue, which ought to be practiced by the manager of every family; but more particularly, at a time when commerce stagnates in our ports, the mechanick is thrown out of employment and the necessaries of life

are so high a price as to be obtained only with the greatest difficulty, and when the poor are precluded altogether from many of them. Every discovery therefore, that has a tendency to ameliorate the condition of the poor and the labourer, and add to their comfort, is of value, and ought to obtain public sanction. The article, coffee, a few years back, was looked upon as unnecessary, but is now considered, from the great use made of it, as one of the necessaries of life. The price is now nearly double to what it was in the year 1811, and continues to rise; a substitute for coffee would therefore be a great object to society in general—many articles have been tried, but, not answering the purpose, have been relinquished. The potatoe is found to resemble coffee in taste, smell and colour, more than any substitute that has been tried; few persons can distinguish one from the other; besides which, it possesses other properties and circumstances which ought to recommend it to general use. It is one of our cheapest and most plentiful vegetables; besides its cheapness, it may be obtained in all places and in any quantity, nore are we dependent on foreign commerce for it—this substitute for coffee sits light on the stomach, is nourishing and easy of digestion, and does not irritate the nerves of weak persons or cause watchfullness. The following is the mode of preparing—Wash raw potatoes clean, cut them into small square pieces, of about the size of a hazel nut; put them into a broad dish or pan, set them in a temperate stove, or in an oven after the bread is taken out, stir them frequently, to prevent them from sticking together, in order that they may dry regularly; when they are perfectly dry, put them into a dry bag or box secure, and they will keep for any length of time.

When they are to be used, they must be roasted or burnt in the same manner as coffee, and ground in a mill or reduced to a powder in a mortar. Small potatoes are as good as the large ones—the potatoes generally considered of the meaner kind are better than the mealy, and the skins and parings are the best of all. It is hoped none will be so prejudiced against this recommendation as not to try it—a trial will confirm what may appear to some to be doubtful.

(*The Farmer's Almanack,* 1815, Boston)

To Make Coffee: Take fresh-roasted coffee, (a quarter of a pound for three persons is the rule, but less will do); allow two tablespoonfuls for each person, grind it just before making, put it in a basin and break into it an egg, yolk, white, shell and all. Mix it up with a spoon to the consistence of mortar, put in warm, not boiling water in the coffee pot; let it boil up and break three times;

then stand a few minutes, and it will be as clear as amber, and the egg will give it a rich taste.

(*Practice of Cookery,* 1830)

BOYS COFFEE: Crumb bread, or dry toast, into a bowl. Put on plenty of sugar, or molasses. Put in one half milk and one half boiling water. To be eaten with a spoon, or drank if preferred. Molasses for sweetening is preferred by most children.

(*Beecher's Receipt Book,* 1857)

These beverages are really delicious and well worth the effort. Go ahead and try a few—you'll never believe how really good soft drinks can be.

Now you'll understand why orangeade became so popular.

ORANGEADE: Squeeze out the juice of an orange, pour boiling water on a little of the peel, and cover it close. Boil water and sugar to a thin syrup, and skim it. When all are cold, mix the juice, the infusion, and the syrup, with as much water as will make a rich drink. Strain through a jelly-bag, and ice.

(*Practical Housewife,* 1860)

This drink enjoyed great popularity. Use sugar cubes in place of the loaf sugar, and regular granulated sugar for the moist.

CAPILLAIRE: Take one pound of loaf sugar, quarter pound of moist sugar, one egg well beaten, one pint of water. Simmer it one hour, skim it while boiling, let it get cold, then boil again and skim, and add one ounce of orange flower water and two tablespoonfuls of brandy. Strain through a jelly-bag, and bottle for use. A spoonful in a tumbler of water makes a pleasant beverage.

(*Godey's Lady's Book,* 1866)

If you're lucky enough to have some currant bushes (or a friend with some), try this drink—it's one of the classics and still a favorite summer refresher in Europe.

CURRANT WATER: Take one pound of currants, and squeeze into a quart of water; put in four or five ounces of powdered sugar. Mix well, strain, and ice or allow to get cold.

This syrup is a nice basic flavoring to have in the cupboard. It makes a very nice beverage when mixed with water or club soda, and is much more wholesome than most of the commercial soft drinks.

ORANGE, OR LEMON SYRUP: Put a pound and a half of white sugar to each pint of juice, add some of the peel, boil ten minutes, then

"The Simple Life"

Consists in observing Nature's laws with untiring fidelity

Kneipp Malt Coffee

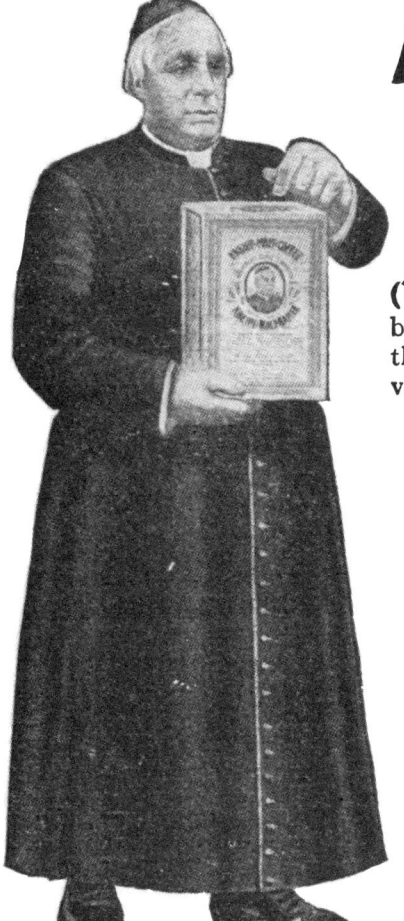

(The **Original Coffee Substitute**) being simplicity itself, is now one of the most noted factors in simple and vigorous living known to mankind.

Its delightful aroma—its appetizing flavor—its nourishing purity—have attracted the world's most talented medical and sanitary experts. The crowned heads and the masses of Europe drink it, and it is fast becoming the favorite family beverage of Americans.

Kneipp Malt Coffee

made only from the purest white Chevalier Malt, cannot possibly contain one atom of adulteration. The Kneipp Malt Food Company has a standing offer of

$1000.00 IN GOLD

to be given to any expert who finds this statement untrue.

Father Sebastian Kneipp's face is to be found on every genuine package.

Would You Like to Test It?

A trial package of Kneipp Malt Coffee and valuable Recipe Book will be sent you, postage prepaid, on receipt of your address and grocer's name, plainly written. Fill out the coupon below and send it to us to-day.

"It's the Way You Make It."
℞ Two tablespoonfuls Kneipp Malt Coffee in one pint of cold water. Add a mere pinch of salt. Let come to a boil, then simmer 6 minutes. Sugar and cream.

Kneipp Malt Food Co.
Box AA, Manitowoc, Wis.

KNEIPP MALT FOOD CO., Manitowoc, Wis.:—Send me trial package of Kneipp Malt Coffee and valuable Recipe Book free of cost and postage prepaid.

Name_____

Street_____ City_____ State_____

Grocer's Name_____

A. S. M.

strain and cork it. It makes a fine beverage, and is useful to flavor pies and puddings.

(*Beecher's Receipt Book,* 1857)

Lemon water is a very light, tart drink—almost like a lemon tea.

LEMON WATER:—is also a delightful drink. Put two slices of lemon, thinly peeled, into a teapot, a little bit of the peel and a large spoonful of capillaire; pour in a pint of boiling water, and stop it close for two hours.

(*Godey's Lady's Book,* 1865)

This is a dessert that never fails to get lots of compliments. Serve it in large wine glasses with a spoon, whether you consider it a beverage or a dessert, it's delicious.

LEMON WATER ICE: Half a pint of lemon-juice, and the same of water, to which put one pint of the syrup of capillaire, the peels of six lemons rubbed off on sugar; strain, mix, and freeze. Then mix up the whites of three eggs to a strong broth, with a little sugar. When the ice is beginning to set, work this well into it, and it will be very soft and delicious.

(*Godey's Lady's Book,* 1866)

The thinner the slices, the more apple flavor you'll end up with. This is a particularly good way to use up those apples that are almost spoiled.

APPLEADE: Cut two large apples in slices, and pour a quart of boiling water on them, strain well and sweeten. To be drunk when cold or iced.

(*Practical Housewife,* 1860)

Habit is a cable. We weave a thread every day, and at last we cannot break it.

(*New England Almanac,* 1840)

Foods

"A small hand will hold only 1½ gills"

In colonial days food was abundant, meals plain but substantial. The housewife set a good table, proud of her cooking and its presentation. A truly native cuisine didn't evolve until the end of the eighteenth century. Up until then the only cooking of any consequence centered around the cultural centers—New York, Boston, Philadelphia, and Virginia. Elsewhere, food was functional and usually mediocre, right up to the early 1800s.

Printed receipt books had a lot to do with the upgrading of American food. Before then receipts were passed via word-of-mouth, often resulting in disasters unless the recipient had an excellent memory and was already an accomplished cook. Even when receipts began to be printed in books, many of their authors felt it was nonsense to specify exact quantities. A perfect example is, "...by practicing the same receipts carefully, the procedures will fix themselves in your mind, so that success is certain. In making pies, for instance, one very heaping handful of flour will make a common-sized pie; not, however, allowing for the flour to be used in rolling the paste. When a woman with an average-sized hand dips it into a flour barrel and comes up with a heaping handful, the amount usually equals ½ pint; contrarily, a small hand will hold only 1½ gills...."

In the receipts I've given amounts are specified; you can therefore be assured of preparing colonial foods that are not only authentic but delicious. I hope you enjoy them. Even if you don't prepare them, they make very interesting reading by showing a side of colonial times that most of us have never seen.

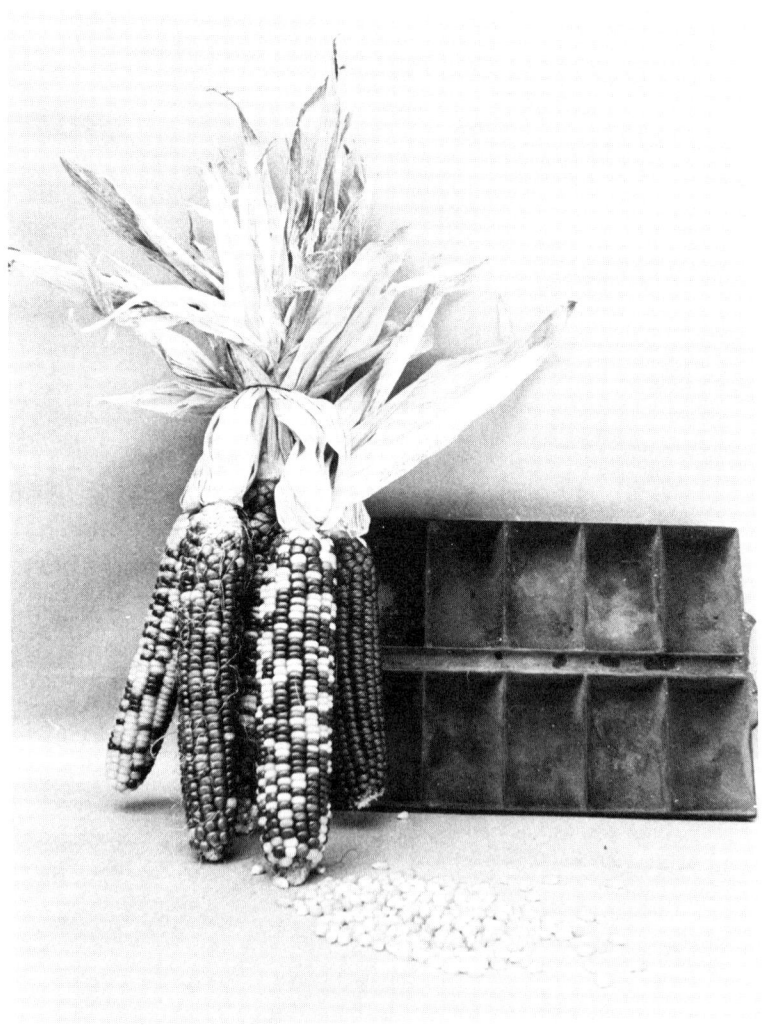

Miscellaneous Rules For The Table

To excite good opinion of the eye, is the first step toward awakening a good appetite. Each dish must be well cooked, and sent to the table, with its proper accompaniment, in the neatest and most elegant manner.

Decoration is most rationally employed in making a plain, nutritious dish inviting.

In preparing dishes for the dinner table, all water should be carefully drained from the vegetables, and the edges of the platters and dishes should be made perfectly clean. All soiled spots should be removed from the outside of gravy boats, or any other article used upon the table. Knives and forks should be clean, and in good order.

In the winter, the comfort of a good meal depends much on having the plates kept warm, and having every dish served hot.

Water should be well drained from cucumbers, greens, and salads. Onions are not as much used as formerly, but when prepared, they are best with fresh meats, and those of a strong flavour, as mutton, goose, and duck.

Jelly is served with mutton, venison, and roasted meats.

Boiled rice looks nice, and is often used with poultry and other meats, as a vegetable, like potatoes.

Fresh pork requires some acid sauce; cranberries or tart applesauce are nice.

Pickles may be served with any meats, but especially with fish. Soy is a fashionable sauce for fish, which is mixed on the plate with drawn butter.

Garnishing dishes, to give them a pleasing look, gives an air of taste and refinement, which is always agreeable.

Stewed fowls, or cold fowl warmed over, look well to have small cups of boiled rice inverted around the edge of the platter, to eat with the meat.

Boiled fish looks neatly with hard-boiled eggs cut in rings, and laid around the edge of the platter, to be served with the fish.

JOIN THE PURE FOOD MOVEMENT

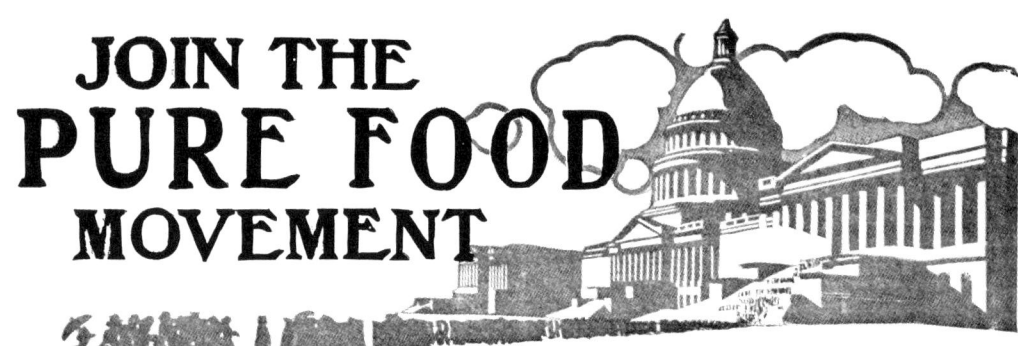

The people have been knocking at the doors of Congress for a pure food law—a law that will protect them from adulterated, misbranded foods.

YOU can join "the pure food movement" NOW, by eating a pure food—a food YOU KNOW is pure and clean—a food that stands the Test of Tooth and Time.

Such a food is shredded whole wheat, made of the best white wheat that grows, cleaned, cooked, drawn into light porous shreds and baked, presenting all the strength-giving elements of the wheat berry in their most digestible form.

The "Tin-Can Age" calls for a Tin-Can Stomach. Have you got one? Don't leave it to Congress. YOU are the "Speaker of the House" in your own home.

Shredded Wheat is not "treated" or "flavored" with anything—not touched by chemicals or human hands—made in the cleanest, finest, most hygienic industrial building on this continent.

Every detail in the process of cleaning, cooking and shredding wheat is open to the world—no "secret process"—nearly 100,000 visitors last year. YOU are invited.

Remember you can grind up "any old thing" and call it a "breakfast food," but you can't SHRED anything but perfect, whole grains of cooked wheat.

THE BISCUIT (warmed in the oven) is delicious for breakfast with hot milk or cream, or for any meal in combination with fresh fruits, creamed meats or vegetables. TRISCUIT is the shredded wheat wafer, used as a Toast with butter, cheese or preserves.

Our new booklets are sent free.

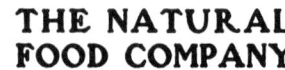

THE NATURAL FOOD COMPANY
Makers of
SHREDDED WHEAT PRODUCTS
Niagara Falls, N. Y.

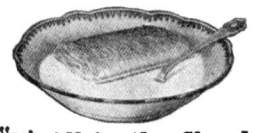

"It's All in the Shreds"

Broiled ham or veal, or fried ham, looks well with boiled eggs, or fried, laid upon each piece.

Asparagus and greens look well laid on buttered toast, with slices of hard-boiled eggs around and on the top, here and there. Common or curled parsley, fastened to the shank of a ham to conceal the bone, and laid around the dish holding it, is a handsome garnish, and looks well around any slices of cold meats, tongue, &c.

The butter should be hard, and made smooth and regular in form or stamped with a figure. It may be made to look neatly with a knife passed over the top after being made smooth, and indenting it with lines.

Bread with meats, if the slices are large, should always be cut in two, and all crumbs removed from the plate, but for tea, left whole.

Cheese should be cut in a thick slice, and then cut in smaller pieces to look neatly.

Custards look neatly, and are better, to be ornamented with a high whip; berries or dots of fine coloured jelly, or cranberry inserted over it, looks well for variety.

Whips on a dessert table look well, and are nice to serve with sweet meats, jellies, and small ripe fruits.

Cake for an evening party looks best to be frosted, and the centre opening filled with a bouquet of flowers. Wreaths of myrtle around those without an opening. Any other simple ornaments that good taste may devise, that are in keeping with the place and occasion, add to the beauty of a table.

(*Etiquette For The Household,* 1855)

Meat & Fish Dishes

Generally the first things that come to mind when we think of colonial food are codfish cakes and Boston baked beans. Cod was certainly a staple for the early settlers (if you remember, the Pilgrims spent their first winter on Cape Cod), and I can't think of any more suitable receipt to start off this section.

CODFISH CAKES: Soak three pounds of salt codfish in cold water till it comes to a boil; pour off the water; if too salt for the taste, add fresh cold water; don't let it boil; when soaked sufficiently remove all the bones and skin and chop fine, boil eight white potatoes till done, draw off the water, mash very fine, add one half-cupful of milk, quarter pound of butter, beat well with a spoon and add to the fish, mixing thoroughly, using more potatoes than fish; roll with the hands into small cakes an inch thick, and fry a rich brown in boiling lard.

(*Peterson's National Ladies Magazine,* 1855)

Here's an old dish that's very good, though not much in favor these days since canned tuna has replaced dried cod.

SALT FISH WITH PARSNIPS: Salt fish must always be well-soaked in plenty of cold water the whole of the night before it is required for the following day's dinner. The salt fish must be put on to boil in plenty of cold water, without any salt, and when thoroughly done, should be well-drained free from any water, and placed on a dish with plenty of well-boiled parsnips. Some sauce may be poured over the fish, which is to be made as follows: Mix two ounces of butter with three ounces of flour, pepper and salt to taste, a small glassful of vinegar and a good half-pint of water. Stir this on the fire till it boils. A few hard-boiled eggs, chopped up and mixed in this sauce, render the dish more acceptable.

(*Ballou's Magazine,* 1850)

You can find out how to roast a turkey in any contemporary cookbook, but I doubt very much you'll find as good a receipt for the colonial's favorite dressing. It's really excellent!

OYSTER DRESSING FOR TURKEY: One lb. of breadcrumbs, two stalks of chopped celery, one-half lb. of butter melted, salt and pepper to taste. Add two quarts of oysters, drained, and carefully looked over for bits of shell. When oysters are mixed with the bread, add enough of the liquor from the oysters to moisten the whole well, and fill with the turkey.

(*McCall's,* December 1870)

This is a very nice change from the usual lobster dishes—it's particularly quick and easy if you use canned lobster.

LOBSTER CUTLETS: Season one pint of chopped lobster meat, with salt, mustard, cayenne, and lemon juice to taste. Moisten with half a pint of thick cream sauce, made by adding one large tablespoonful of butter, two large tablespoonfuls of flour seasoned with a little salt and pepper, and pouring on a cupful of hot milk. Cool, shape into cutlets, dip in breadcrumbs, in beaten egg and again in crumbs, and fry in fat hot enough to brown bread while counting fifty. Garnish with parsley and serve with sauce.

(*McCall's,* December 1875)

This receipt makes a nice, basic cold meat salad. You can use any type of cold meat, fowl or fish—the variations are limitless.

VEAL SALAD: Cut cold roast veal or stewed veal into small pieces. Cut in very small thin bits with a sharp knife as much cold boiled potatoes as you have meat; place lettuce leaves around a flat dish, place meat and potatoes in a heap in the centre after mixing a good mayonnaise through it. Season with salt and pepper to taste. Cut slices of cold boiled egg on top and pour over a little more mayonnaise.

(*Household Receipts,* 1852)

This is a very nice change from duck with orange sauce, and a good deal easier. Since today's ducks are very fatty I would omit the bacon and the basting with butter.

ROAST DUCK: Pluck, singe, and draw; blanch the feet, and remove their skin; make a stuffing with sage, onions (previously blanched and chopped fine), and bread-crumbs, using twice as much onion as sage, and twice as much bread-crumbs as onion; add a little butter, pepper, and salt to taste. When stuffed, truss; tie some slices of bacon over the breasts; roast for fifteen minutes before a brisk fire, then move away and roast until done. Remove the bacon a minute or two before they are roasted. Serve with gravy in the dish, but not over the birds.

(*Peterson's National Ladies Magazine,* July 1865)

This is a very flavorful method for roasting veal. It's surprising how much difference a bit of lemon juice makes.

ROAST VEAL: Take from four to six pounds of the best end of the

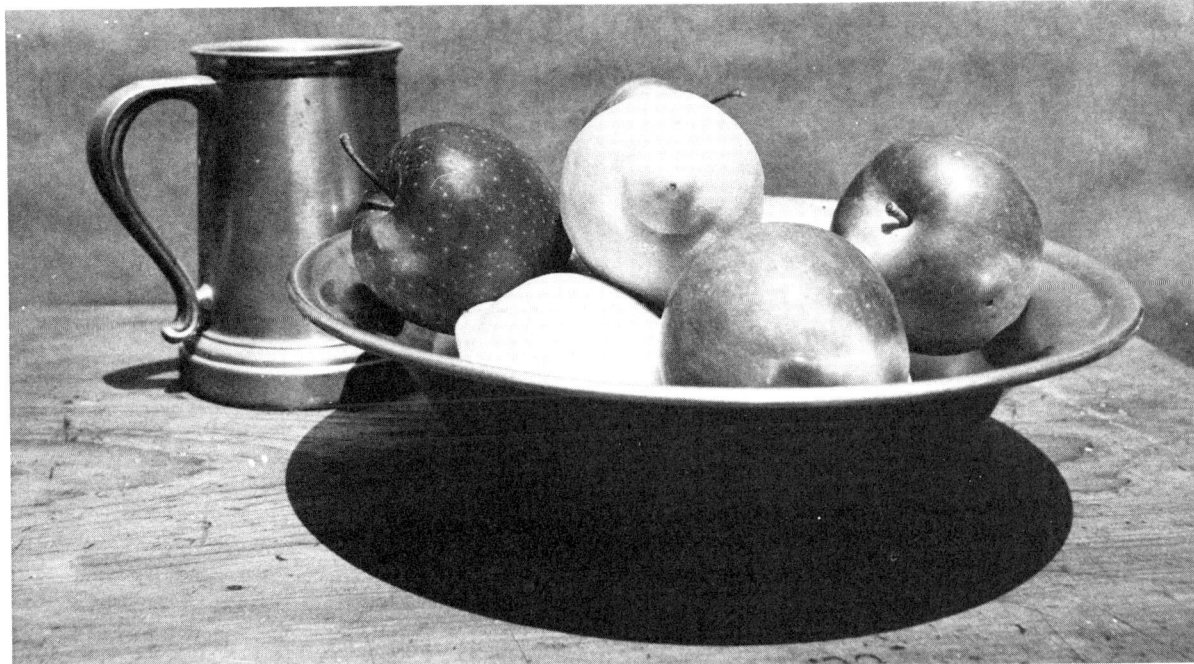

neck of veal, trim it neatly, and joint. Put it to roast at a very moderate fire, and baste it plentifully every ten minutes, first with butter, and then with its own gravy. It will take from one and a-half to more than two hours. During the last quarter of an hour, bring the joint nearer the fire, and sprinkle it plentifully with salt. Serve with the gravy over, carefully strained and freed from fat, and with the juice of a lemon and a small piece of fresh butter added to it.

(*Ladies Cabinet,* 1873)

These needn't be mutton chops (which incidentally are next to impossible to find these days), but any cut of pork or lamb will do. Use an inexpensive cut, in any case. And you can always use a piecrust mix if the mysteries of pastry making elude you....

MEAT PIE: Season mutton chops (those from the neck are best) pretty highly with pepper and salt, and place them in a dish in layers, with plenty of sliced apples, sweetened and chopped onions; cover with a good suet crust, and bake. When done, pour out all the gravy at the side, take off the fat, and add a spoonful of mushroom ketchup [see glossary], then return it to the pie. The apples may be omitted or not according to the taste.

(*Household Discoveries,* 1845)

This is just about as all-American as you can get!

BEEFSTEAK SMOTHERED IN ONIONS: Take a juicy beefesteak two inches thick; broil it nicely, then have ready six onions, sliced and fried in butter; be careful not to let them burn; fry them a light brown. When the steak is done and ready to serve, put several lumps of butter upon it, and pour two tablespoonfuls of boiling water over it; then pour on the hot onions, and serve immediately. The onions should be allowed to lie in salt-and-water for an hour, and then wiped dry before putting them into the butter to fry.

(*Peterson's National Ladies Magazine,* October 1854)

Simply delicious!

HASHED FOWL: Take the meat from a cold fowl and cut into small pieces. Put half-a-pint of well-flavored stock into a stewpan, add a little salt, pepper, and nutmeg, and thicken with some flour and butter; let it boil, then put in the pieces of fowl to warm; after warming sufficiently, serve with some poached eggs laid on the hash, with a sprig of parsley in the centre, and garnish round the plate with pieces of fried bread.

(*The Practical Housekeeper,* 1870)

This is an excellent way to use up any small pieces of leftover meat. If you have the time, run them under the broiler just long enough to brown them very lightly.

COLD TONGUE ON TOAST: Take cold smoked tongue or ham, mince or grate fine, mix it with the beaten yolk of an egg and cream or milk, with a dash of cayenne pepper; prepare small, thin round or square pieces of buttered toast; place on a heated platter, putting a spoonful of meat on each piece; cover with a dish-cover, and send to the table hot; for breakfast or lunch.

(*The Ladies Companion,* 1873)

Rabbit isn't often for sale on the meat counters these days, but if you check the frozen food cases in the large supermarket chains you'll probably be able to find frozen rabbit pieces. The flavor is very much like chicken and many people find they really like it.

RABBIT STEWED WITH CABBAGE: Trim off the stalk and outside leaves of a fresh young cabbage. Cut into four, wash it, and leave it in cold water. Cut up the rabbit into joints; season with a teaspoonful of pepper, a saltspoonful of salt, and the same of mace. Cut up a pound of the thick part of pickled pork into short slices a quarter of an inch thick; trim, wash, and cut up two large leeks. Put the whole, except the cabbage, into a saucepan, with just enough water to cover the rabbit. Boil up slowly. Put in the cabbage; press it down well into the gravy, and continue to simmer without the lid for another hour, or till the cabbage is tender; press the cabbage down often. Serve the whole in the same dish.

(*Ballou's Magazine,* 1861)

Another great way to use up leftover meat.

COLD MINCED MEAT AND EGGS: Take some fragments of any cold roast meat. Trim off all the fat parts and mince it very finely. Fry a shallot chopped small in plenty of butter; when it is light brown add a large pinch of flour and a little stock, then add the minced meat, with chopped parsley, pepper, salt, and nutmeg to taste. Mix well, add a little more stock, if necessary, and let the mince gradually get hot by the side of the fire; lastly drop in a few drops of lemon juice; serve with sippets of bread fried in butter; and place a poached egg on top.

(*The Christian Herald & Signs Of Our Times,* April 1861)

A really great method for baking ham...

BAKED HAM: Make a thick paste of flour and water (not boiled) and cover the entire ham with it, bone and all; put it in a pan or spider on two muffin rings, or anything else that will keep it an inch from the bottom, and bake in a hot oven; if a small ham, fifteen minutes for each pound; if large twenty minutes; the oven should be hot when put in. The paste forms the hard crust around the ham, and the skin comes off with it. Try this and you will never cook a ham in any other way.

(*Household Discoveries,* 1863)

Sweetbreads are one of my favorite meat dishes, and this receipt is an excellent way to prepare them, especially if you've never tried them before.

TOMATO SWEETBREADS: Cut up a quarter of a peck of fine ripe tomatoes; set them over the fire and let them stew in nothing but their own juices till they go to pieces—then strain them through a sieve; have ready four or five sweetbreads that have been trimmed nicely and soaked in warm water. Put them into a stewpan with the tomato juice, and a little salt and cayenne; add two or three tablespoons butter rolled in flour. Set the saucepan over the fire, and stew the sweetbreads until done. A few minutes before you take them up, stir in two beaten yolks of eggs. Serve the sweetbreads in a deep dish, with the tomato sauce poured over them.

(*Mrs. Winslow's Domestic Receipt Book,* 1855)

Here's another receipt for sweetbreads that's absolutely scrumptious!

SWEETBREADS AND CAULIFLOWERS: Take four large sweetbreads and two cauliflowers. Split open the sweetbreads and remove the gristle. Soak them awhile in lukewarm water; put them into a saucepan of boiling water, and set them to boil ten minutes. Afterwards lay them in a pan of cold water to make them firm. The parboiling is to whiten them. Wash, drain, and quarter the cauliflowers. Put them in a broad stewpan with the sweetbreads on them; season with a little nutmeg and a little cayenne—add water to cover them. Put on the lid of the pan and stew one hour. Take a quarter of a pound of fresh butter and roll it in two teaspoonfuls of flour; add this with a teacup of milk to the stew, and give it one boil up and no more. Serve hot, in a deep dish. This stew will be found delicious.

(*Mrs. Abell's Receipts,* 1840)

Another variation on the shepherd's pie—sort of an old-fashioned version of Hamburger Helper.

AN ECONOMICAL DISH: Steam or boil some mealy potatoes; mash them together with some butter or cream, season them, and place a

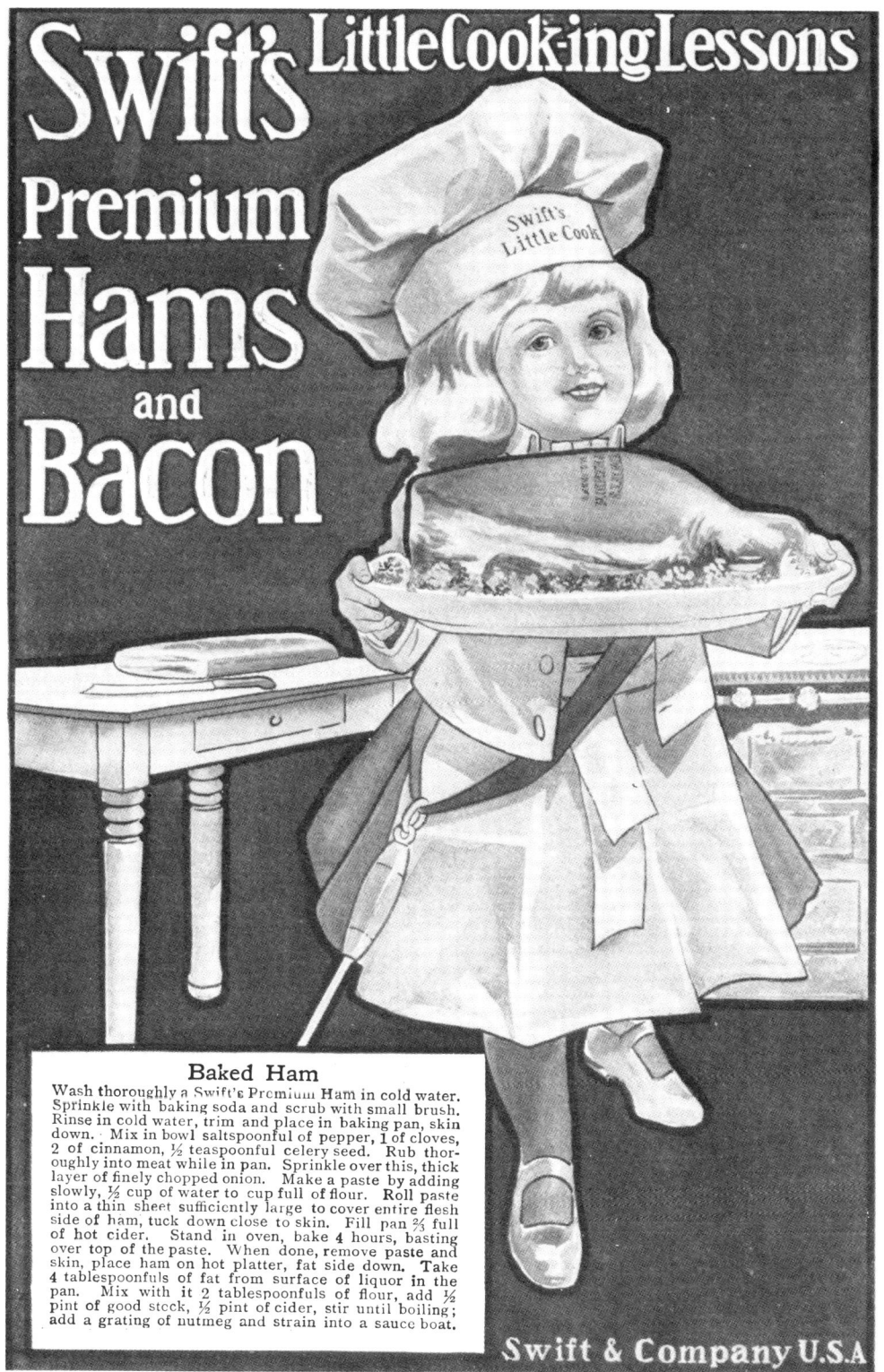

layer at the bottom of the pie-dish; upon this place a layer of finely chopped cold meat or fish of any kind, well-seasoned; then add another layer of potatoes, and continue alternating these with more chopped meat until the dish is filled. Smooth down the top, strew breadcrumbs upon it; and bake until it is brown. A very small quantity of meat serves in this manner to make a nice, presentable little dish. A sprinkling of chopped pickles may be added, if convenient, and when fish is employed, it eats better if first beaten up with raw eggs.

(*The Mother's Book Of Daily Duties,* 1855)

Even as far back as 1840 they were thinking up fancy names for simple everyday stews! This can be varied by adding potatoes, carrots, celery, or whatever vegetables you have on hand—and canned tomatoes will substitute very nicely for the ripe ones.

FRENCH STEW: Cut into pieces two or three pounds of the lean of fresh, tender beef, veal or pork, and peel and slice a quarter of a peck of ripe tomatoes; season the whole with a little salt and pepper. Put the whole into a stew pot, and cover it close, opening it only occasionally to see how it is cooking. Put no water to stew, the juice of the tomatoes is enough liquid. When the tomatoes are all dissolved, stir in a piece of fresh butter dredged with flour. Let it stew about a quarter of an hour longer. When the meat is done through, have ready some bits of very dry toast cut in three-cornered shape, leaving the crust off. Dip the toast for a moment in some hot water, butter it, and stand it up around the inside of a deep dish. Fill in the stew and serve hot.

(*Domestic Receipts,* 1840)

These will keep uncooked in the refrigerator for four or five days. I usually make the receipt with half a pound of pork, half a pound of veal, a quarter pound of suet, and about one-third of a cup of breadcrumbs. If you like, a bit of minced garlic is very good.

OXFORD SAUSAGES: Chop one and one-half pounds pork, one and one-half pounds of veal, free from skin, etc., three-fourths of a pound of beef suet; mince and mix well, stir the crumb of a penny-loaf in water, mix with the meat. Add sage, salt, pepper and allspice to taste. Roll into balls, flatten, and fry of a light brown.

(*Mrs. Winslow's Domestic Receipt Book,* 1868)

A really delicious way to stretch seafood. Serve with lemon slices, your favorite seafood sauce, or plain. They'll be delectable any way you choose.

LOBSTER RISSOLES: Extract the meat of a boiled lobster; mince it as finely as possible; mix it with the coral pounded smooth, and some yolks of hard-boiled eggs, pounded also. Season it with Cayenne pepper, powdered mace, and a very little salt. Make a batter of beaten egg, milk, and flour. To each egg allow two large tablespoonfuls of milk, and a large tablespoonful of flour. Beat the batter well, and then mix the lobster with it gradually, till it is stiff enough to make into oval balls about the size of a large plum. Fry them in the best salad oil, and serve them up either warm or cold. Similar rissoles may be made of raw oysters minced fine, or raw clams. These should be fried in lard.

(*Mrs. Winslow's Domestic Receipt Book,* 1870)

Oysters were a great favorite in colonial times; the following is a method the colonists devised to keep oysters fresh until they were needed.

TO KEEP OYSTERS: After washing them, lay them in a tub with the deep part of the shell undermost, sprinkle them with salt and Indian meal, or flour, fill the tub with cold water, and set in a cool place. Change the water daily, and they will keep fresh a fortnight.

(*Mrs. Abell's Receipts,* 1845)

And now that you have oysters in the pantry, here are two excellent ways to use them up.

TO FRY OYSTERS: Make a batter, as for pancakes; put one or two oysters into a spoonful of the batter, and fry them to a light brown. Fry them in hot fat, the same as pancakes.

STEWED OYSTERS: Three quarts are enough for a small family dinner. Put them into a saucepan, with a piece of butter the size of an egg; stew them well ten minutes; toast three or four slices of bread, cut them, lay them in the botton of the dish, and pour the oysters over them.

(*The Married Ladies' Indispensable Companion & Family Physician,* 1850)

A simple lobster soup, basically made the same way as an oyster stew. Use leftover or canned lobster meat and, if possible, use Half & Half in place of the milk.

LOBSTER SOUP: After having boiled the lobster, take it from the shell, roll two or three crackers, and put it to the meat, which may be cut up small; melt some butter in a stew-pan, two quarts of boiling milk or water, and salt and pepper to taste: let it boil gently

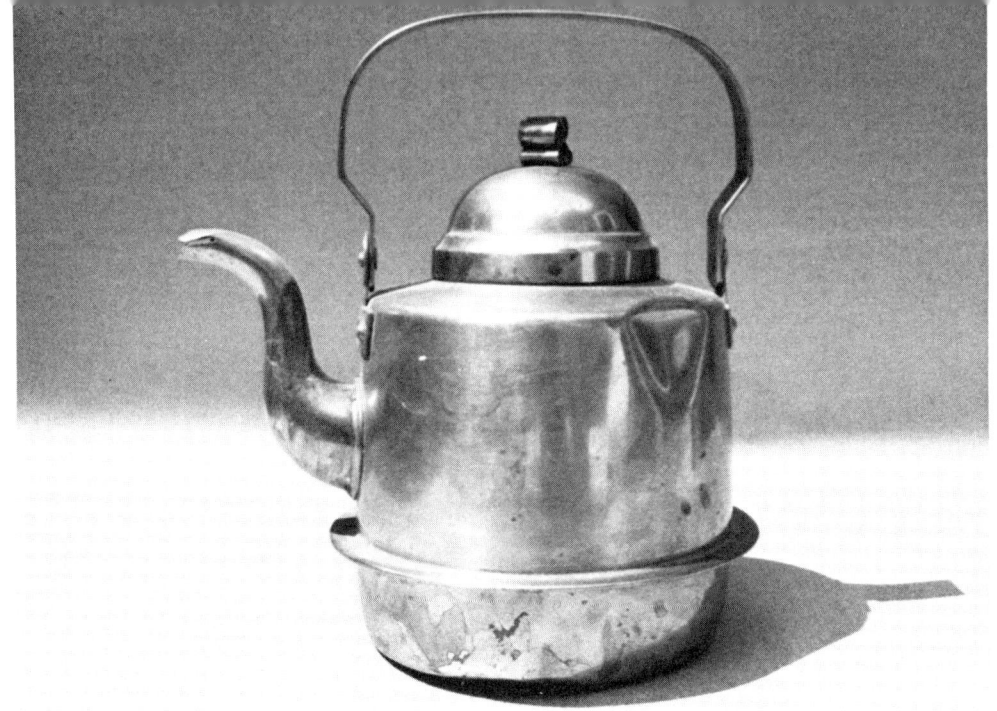

for fifteen minutes; put some crackers in a tureen; pour over the soup, and serve.

(*Mrs. Abell's Receipts,* 1845)

A genuine old-fashioned chowder. Add or delete from this receipt to suit your own needs and taste. I add onion and substitute milk for the water.

TO MAKE A CHOWDER: Cut three or four slices of fat pork; fry them a very little; lay them in the bottom of a stew-kettle. Cut a fresh cod into thin slices; place two slices of fish on the pork; then put in a layer of split crackers; pare and wash eight potatoes, and cut them into thin slices; put on a layer of the sliced potatoes, then alternately the other materials, till the kettle is full; season with pepper and a little salt. Mix one table-spoonful of flour with a tea-cupful of cold water, and pour in after the chowder begins to stew. Put in a quart of water, cover the stew-kettle very tight, and let it stew three hours.

(*Household Receipts,* 1840)

I must admit it's an almost impossible feat to find the turtle, but if you manage to find one you'll know what to do with it!

TURTLE SOUP: Cut the head off the turtle the day before you dress it, and place the body so as to drain it well from blood; the next day cut it up in the following manner: Divide the back, belly, fins, and head from the intestines and lean parts; take care to cut the gall clean out without breaking, scald in boiling water the first named parts, so as to take off the skin and shell; cut them in pieces small enough to stew, and throw them in cold water; boil the back and the belly in water long enough to extract the bones; put the meat on a dish, then make a good stock of a leg of veal, lean ham and the flesh of the inside of the turtle; draw it down to a colour, then fill it up with beef stock, and the liquor and the bones of the boiled turtle. Season with stalks of marjoram, and boil some onions, a bunch of parsley, cloves and whole pepper. Let it boil slowly for four hours, then strain it to the pieces of back, fins, belly, and head of the turtle; take the bones from the fins, and cut the rest in neat, square pieces with as little waste as possible.—Thicken the stock with butter rolled in flour, and boil it, to cleanse it from grease and scum; then strain it through a cloth—then boil your herbs that have been washed and pickled, in a bottle of Madeira wine with a little sugar.—The herbs that have to be used are marjoram, thyme, basil, and parsley; then put together soup, meat, herbs, and some force meat; and egg-balls. Boil it a short time, and put it away in clean pans until the following day, as the rawness will go off, and the flavour be improved by so doing. In cutting up the turtle meat the fat should be taken great care of. It should be separated, cut in neat pieces, and stewed tender in a little of the soup, and put in the tureen at last.

(*Valuable Receipts,* 1860)

And while you're searching for the turtle you can make this version which doesn't require any turtle meat....

MOCK TURTLE SOUP: Take one pound and a half of lean veal, or tripe (which is best), cut it into small slices, and fry to a delicate brown. Cut the meat from three cow-heels in tolerably large pieces, then put it with the fried veal or tripe into a pint and a half of weak gravy, with three anchovies, a little salt, some cayenne pepper, three blades of mace, nine cloves, the green parts of three leeks, three sprigs of lemon thyme, some parsley and lemon peel; chop these last very fine before adding them; let the whole stew gently for three hours—then squeeze the juice of three lemons to it; add three glasses of Madeira wine, and let it stew for one hour more,—then skim off the fat, and serve.

(*The Married Ladies' Indispensable Companion & Family Physician,* 1850)

A very pleasant dish, especially if you enjoy pickled fish. It's great either as an appetizer or first course.

FRESH MACKEREL SOUSED: After having thoroughly cleaned them, boil them in salt water until tender; then take them out, lay them in a deep dish; take of the water in which they were boiled, half as much as will cover them; add to it as much more vinegar, some whole pepper, cloves, and a blade or two of mace. Pour it over hot; in two days it will be fit to eat.

(*Valuable Receipts,* 1860)

A soup derived from the New England Boiled Dinner. Nourishing and filling on a cold fall evening, easy to prepare, and truly American.

CABBAGE SOUP: Boil corned beef in a pot of water till half done, then add two small heads of cabbage cut in quarters, and well washed (examine carefully, as insects are sometimes concealed between the leaves); when it is done tender, take out the largest pieces and drain them in a cullender, and set it over a pot of hot water to keep it hot; if the meat is tender, take that up also, and add to the soup a cup of pearl barley or rice, a dozen or more potatoes peeled and cut in half; two or three turnips and some sliced or grated carrots—if liked, an onion or two may be added; let it boil until the vegetables are all done; put the meat on a large dish, and the cabbage and other vegetables on small dishes, for side dishes. This makes a good family dinner. Serve the soup in tureen hot; thicken with a table-spoonful of flour made in thin paste with water.

(*Domestic Receipts,* 1840)

A very basic version of chicken soup. If you can possibly get one, a chicken marked "fowl" is superior to the commonly available "fryer" or "broiler."

CHICKEN SOUP: An old fowl makes good soup. Cut it up—first take off the wings, legs, and neck, then divide it down the sides, and cut the back and breast each in two pieces; cut half a pound of pork in thin slices, and put it with the cut-up fowl into four or five pints of water; set it over gentle fire, skim it clear, taking care not to keep it open longer than is necessary; add a cup of rice or pearl-barley, cayenne or black pepper to taste, a leek sliced, and potatoes cut in half—if liked, a grated or sliced carrot, and a turnip cut small may be added.

(*Household Discoveries,* 1863)

Use neck of lamb in place of the mutton. You're probably best acquainted with this soup as Scotch Broth.

MUTTON BROTH: Take a neck of mutton, cut it in pieces, reserving a good-sized piece to serve in the tureen; put it in cold water enough to cover it, and cover the pot close; set it on coals until the water is lukewarm, then pour it off, and skim it well; then put it again to the

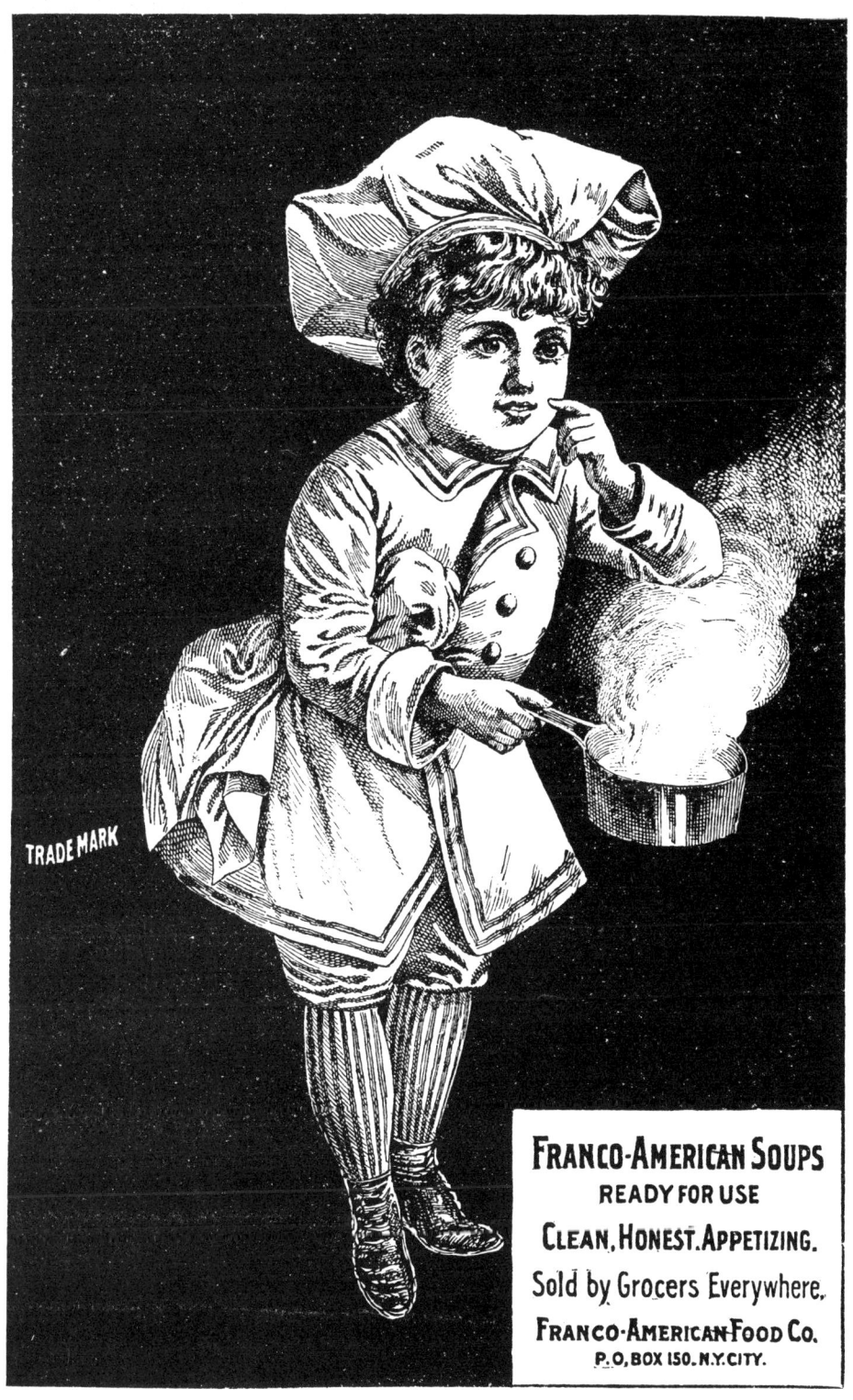

meat with the addition of five pints of water, a tea-spoonful of rice or pearl barley, and an onion cut up; set it on a slow fire, and when you have taken all the scum off, put in two or three quartered turnips. Let it simmer very slowly for two hours, then strain it through a sieve into the tureen; add pepper and salt to taste.

(Married Ladies' Indispensable Companion & Home Physician, 1850)

Still considered a great gourmet treat, roast suckling pig is quite a culinary presentation. Much more common in colonial times when everyone raised their own, it's still worth the effort for a large buffet. Oh, don't forget the traditional garnish of a brightly polished red apple in the mouth!

TO ROAST A PIG: A pig about three weeks old is the best. It should be killed in the morning, if it is to be eaten for dinner. Make a stuffing with about six powdered crackers, one table-spoonful of sage, two of sweet marjoram, half a pint of cream, two eggs, and a little salt and pepper. Mix these well together, and let it stew about fifteen minutes. Wash the pig in cold water; cut off the petti-toes, leaving the skin long enough to wrap around the ends of the legs; then fill the belly with stuffing, and sew it up. The liver and the heart should be boiled with five or six peppercorns, and chopped fine for the gravy. When the pig is put down to roast, put in a pint of water, and a table-spoonful of salt; when it begins to roast, flour it well, and baste it with the drippings and continue to do so until it is done. It requires constant care. A small pig will roast in three hours.

(Married Ladies' Indispensable Companion & Home Physician, 1850)

A nice change from packaged sausages. Use your meat grinder and it's no effort at all.

SAUSAGE MEAT: Chop two pounds of lean beef, with one of fat pork, very fine; mix it with three tea-spoonfuls of salt, five of powdered sage, five of sweet marjoram, three of black pepper. Make this into small cakes, and fry in the same manner as sausages, is very good for breakfast.

(Valuable Receipts, 1860)

A good honest chicken pot pie without unnecessary vegetables or other adornments. For the crust I use biscuit dough rolled a quarter of an inch thick.

CHICKEN POT PIE: Wash and cut the chicken into joints; take out the breast bone; boil them about twenty minutes; take them up;

wash out your kettle; fry two or three slices of fat salt pork, and put in the bottom of the kettle; then put in the chicken, with about three pints of water, a piece of butter the size of an egg; sprinkle in a teaspoonful of pepper, and cover over the top with a light crust. It will require an hour to cook.

(*Valuable Receipts,* 1860)

There's not much I can say that the name of this receipt doesn't say better.

A VERY GOOD WAY TO PREPARE CHICKEN; Wash, and cut the chicken into joints; scald, and take off the skin; put the pieces in a stew-pan, with very little parsley, thyme, salt and pepper; add a quart of water, and a piece of butter the size of an egg; stew it an hour and a half; take up the chicken, and if there is no gravy, add another piece of butter, very little water, and sprinkle in a tablespoonful of flour, and let it boil ten mintues.

(*Peterson's National Ladies Magazine,* 1860)

A great way to use up cold steak.

BEEF BALLS: Mince very finely a piece of tender cooked beef, fat and lean, mince an onion, with some parsley; add grated bread crumbs, and season with pepper, salt, grated nutmeg, and lemon-peel; mix all together, and moisten it with an egg beaten; roll it into balls, flour and fry them in boiling fresh dripping. Serve them with fried bread crumbs, or with thickened brown gravy.

(*Valuable Receipts,* 1860)

Nice simple suggestions on how to cook sweet breads, livers and hearts.

SWEET BREAD, LIVER, AND HEART: A very good way to cook the sweet bread is to fry three or four slices of pork till brown, then take them up and put in the sweet bread, and fry it over a medium fire. When you have taken up the sweet bread, mix a couple of teaspoonfuls of flour with a little water, and stir it into the fat. Let it boil, then turn it over the sweet bread. Another way is to parboil them, and let them get cold, then, cut them in pieces about an inch thick, dip them in the yolk of an egg, and fine bread crumbs, sprinkle salt, pepper, and sage on them, before dipping them in the egg, fry them a light brown. Make a gravy after you have taken them up, by stirring a little flour and water mixed smooth into the fat, add spices and wine if you like. The liver and heart are good cooked in the same manner, or broiled.

(*The Married Ladies' Indispensable Companion & Family Physician,* 1850)

Sort of the original inspiration for the bouillon cube.

PORTABLE SOUP: This is a very good and nutritious soup, made first into jelly and then congealed into hard cakes, resembling glue. If well made, it will keep for many months in a cool dry place and when dissolved in water or gravy will afford a fine liquid soup, very convenient to carry on a journey or sea voyage, or to use in a remote place where meat for soup is not to be had. A piece of this glue the size of a large walnut will, when melted down in water, become a pint bowl of soup; or by using less water you may have it much richer. If there is time and opportunity, boil with the piece of soup a seasoning of sliced onion, sweet marjoram, sweet basil, or any herbs you choose. Also, a bit of butter rolled in flour.

To make portable soup, take two shins or legs of beef, two knuckles of veal, and four unskinned calf's feet. Have the bones broken or cracked. Have the whole put in a large clean pot that will hold four gallons of water. Pour in, at the beginning, only as much water as will cover the meat well and set it over the fire so that it will heat gradually till it almost boils. Watch and skim carefully while any scum rises. Then throw in a quart of cold water to make it throw up all the remaining scum, and then let come to a complete boil, continuing to skim as long as any scum appears. In this be particular. When the liquid appears clear and completely free from grease, pour in the remainder of the water and let it boil very gently for eight hours. Strain it through a very clean hair sieve into a large stoneware pan and let it cool quickly. Next day remove all the grease and pour the liquid as quickly as possible into a three-gallon stew pan, taking care not to disturb the settlings at the bottom. Keep the pan uncovered and let boil as quickly as possible over a quick fire. Next transfer it to a three-quart stew pan and skim it again if necessary. Watch it well and see that it does not burn, for that would spoil the whole. Take out a little in a spoon and hold it in the air to see if it will jelly. If it will not, boil a little longer. Till it jellies it is not done. Have ready some small whiteware preserve pots clean and quite dry. Fill them with the soup and let them stand, undisturbed, until the next day. Set over a slow fire a large flat-bottomed stew pan, one third filled with boiling water. Place in it the pots of soup, seeing it does not reach within two inches of the rims. Let the pots stand uncovered in this water, hot, but not boiling, for six or seven hours. This will bring the soup to a proper thickness, which should be that of a stiff jelly when hot, and when cold it should be like hard glue. When finished turn out the molds of soup, and wrap them up in clean brownish paper, and put them up in boxes, breaking off a piece when wanted to dissolve this soup. Portable soup may be improved by the additions of three pounds of nice lean beef, to the shins, knuckles and calf's feet, &c. If you have any friends going the overland journey, to the Pacific a box of this portable soup may be a most useful present to them.

(*Miss Leslie's Receipts*, 1857)

Vegetables & Sauces

A very sophisticated potato dish that is still very popular in French cookbooks. The trick to getting these to puff properly is to make sure the fat is *very* hot—almost smoking—the second time you deep-fry them.

SOUFFLEED POTATOES: Peel potatoes, cut them, in the direction of their length, into slices a quarter of an inch thick, fry them until they are three parts done, in moderately hot fat. Take them out, drain, and let nearly get cold. Throw them into very hot fat, and plenty of it; keep them moving with a spoon until they are well souffleed or swollen, and of a light-brown, which takes place almost immediately.

(*Peterson's National Ladies Magazine*, August 1860)

A fabulous way to fix green beans that aren't as tender as they might be.

HARICOT BEANS WITH TOMATOES: Take a quantity of fresh haricot beans, being careful to get them all of an age. Boil them in plenty of salted water. Drain when done, and add to them as much tomatoe sauce as they will take, and also some fine minced parsley.

(*Ladies Gazette*, 1859)

Delicious on a cold fall day, and still another way to use up leftovers.

POTATOE PUFF: Take cold roast meat—beaf or mutton, or veal and ham together—clear from gristle, cut small, and season with pepper and salt, and cut pickles, if desired. Boil and mash some potatoes, make them into a paste with an egg, and roll out, dredging with flour. Cut round with a saucer; put some of the seasoned meat upon one-half, and fold over the other half like a puff; pinch neatly round, and fry light-brown. This is a good method of warming up meat which has been cooked.

(*Ballou's Magazine*, 1841)

Make this with salmon, garnish with some fresh herbs, and you'll have a truly impressive salad for the most enjoyable summer buffet imaginable!

POTATOE SALAD & SALAD DRESSING: Cut a dozen cold boiled potatoes into fancy shapes, one-quarter of an inch thick; mix with some flakes of cold boiled fish—halibut, cod, or salmon—and pour over them a boiled dressing, made with six tablespoonfuls of melted butter or olive oil, six tablespoonfuls of cream or milk, one teaspoonful of salt, half that quantity of pepper, and one teaspoonful of ground mustard. Into this mix one small cupful of vinegar. Boil well; then add three eggs beaten to a foam; remove directly from the fire and stir for five minutes. When thoroughly cold, turn over the salad, garnish with slices of pickled cucumbers, beet-root, hard-boiled eggs, and fresh parsley. This boiled salad can be made in quantities, and kept bottled for weeks. It is very palatable. When used for green salads it should be placed at the bottom of the bowl, and the salad on top; for if mixed, the vegetables lose that crispness which is so delicious to the epicure.

(*Peterson's National Ladies Magazine,*
July 1860)

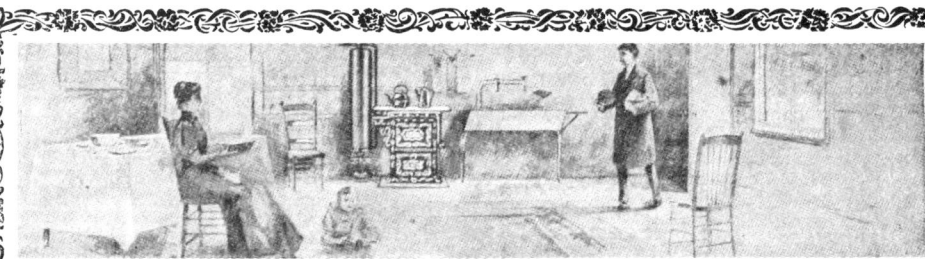

Cooking by Gas
Costs less than Cooking by Coal or Wood;

and how much easier and quicker is the process. No smoke, no soot, no ashes or litter, no sweltering heat; a match builds the fire, a slight movement of the hand extinguishes it. Of course, much depends on the stove, and there is only one Gas Stove that combines the greatest economy with the highest efficiency and convenience. That's the . . .

A Stove that's made in "the Largest and Best-Equipped Stove-Plant in the World." . . . .

Detroit Jewel.

THIS TRADE-MARK APPEARS ON EVERY DETROIT JEWEL.

Write for a copy of our "Cooking by Gas." An up-to-date pamphlet for up-to-date housekeepers. Contains a chapter of Choice Cooking Recipes. *Please mention Harper's Magazine.*

JEWEL STOVES AND RANGES
LARGEST STOVE PLANT IN THE WORLD

Detroit, Mich.   DETROIT STOVE WORKS.   Chicago, Ill.

A nice, creamy dressing to which you can add any number of other ingredients to vary it to your taste. I like it with some finely minced fresh tarragon over cold chicken.

SALAD DRESSING: One teaspoonful of made mustard, one teaspoonful of sugar, two tablespoonfuls of olive oil, a tablespoonful of milk or cream, two of vinegar, cayenne pepper and salt to taste. Put the mustard into a salad bowl with the sugar, and add the oil drop by drop, carefully stirring and mixing all the ingredients well-together. Proceed in this manner with the milk and vinegar, which must be added very gradually or the sauce will curdle; then put in the seasoning of cayenne and salt. It ought to have a creamy appearance and when mixing, the ingredients cannot be added too gradually, or stirred too much.

(*Household Discoveries,* 1854)

Here's another cooked dressing that uses butter rather than oil.

CREAM DRESSING FOR SALAD: Beat together thoroughly three raw eggs and six tablespoonfuls of cream, three tablespoonfuls of melted butter, one teaspoonful of salt, one of mustard, one-half of black pepper, and one teacup of vinegar. Heat, stirring it constantly, until it thickens like boiled custard. If it boils, it will curdle. Let it cool, then mix with salad.

(*Peterson's National Ladies Magazine,*
August 1849)

This sure beats commercially bottled mint sauce and it's so easy to make there's no reason not to enjoy it!

MINT SAUCE: Chop as finely as possible a quantity of mint leaves previously washed; add to these sufficient vinegar and water, in equal parts, to float them, add a small quantity of powdered sugar. Let the sauce stand for an hour before serving.

(*Ballou's Magazine,* 1847)

A beautiful rich green sauce that adds color to otherwise plain dishes. If you enjoy the flavor of parsley you can use two or three tablespoonfuls without altering the rest of the receipt.

PARSLEY SAUCE: Boil a pint of water, throw into it a tablespoonful of finely minced parsley and a half-teaspoonful of salt, then stir two ounces of flour mixed smooth in a gill of cold water. Stir over the fire till it thickens, break into it one or two ounces of butter, and, as soon as it is melted, serve the sauce.

MAITRE D'HOTEL SAUCE: Make as above, and when the sauce is

taken off the fire, add the juice of half a lemon. If the acid is allowed to boil with the parsley, it will spoil the colour.

(Peterson's National Ladies Magazine, October 1870)

This will probably seem a silly receipt to some, but the difference between a properly cooked potato and one that has been haphazardly prepared is incredible.

To Boil Potatoes: In the best manner, is a great perfection in cooking. The following way is a good one. Take potatoes as equal in size as possible; wash, but do not pare or cut them; put them into a pot, the largest potatoes at the bottom; cover them with cold water, about an inch over; too much water injures them very much; throw in a spoonful of salt, and let them boil about five minutes; then take off the pot, and set it where it will simmer slowly for thirty minutes; then try the potatoes with a fork; if it pass easily through they are done; if not, let them simmer until they are; then pour off the water; place the pot where the potatoes will keep hot, but not burn, and let them stand uncovered till the moisture shall have evaporated. They will then be mealy and in perfection. Potatoes, either boiled or roasted, should *never* be covered to keep them hot.

(Valuable Receipts, 1855)

The addition of milk to the water in which onions are cooked makes a delightful difference.

Onions: Peel them and put them into boiling milk and water, (water alone will do, but it is not so good). When tender, take them up, and salt them, and turn a little melted butter over them.

(Peterson's National Ladies Magazine, August 1881)

A great way to vary mashed potatoes.

Onion Ormoloo: Peel ten or twelve large white onions, steep them an hour in cold water, then boil them till soft. Mash them with an equal quantity of boiled potatoes, adding half a pint of milk and two or three well-beaten eggs.—Stir the mixture very hard, season it with nutmeg, pepper and salt, and bake in a quick oven; when half done pour a little melted butter or gravy over the top.

(Mrs. Winslow's Domestic Receipt Book, 1870)

This receipt can be made using just about any variety of dried beans; I use navy or lentils. A touch of sherry or Madeira improves the flavor.

Bean Soup: Wash and boil your beans with a piece of salt pork. When the beans are soft take them out, and press through a

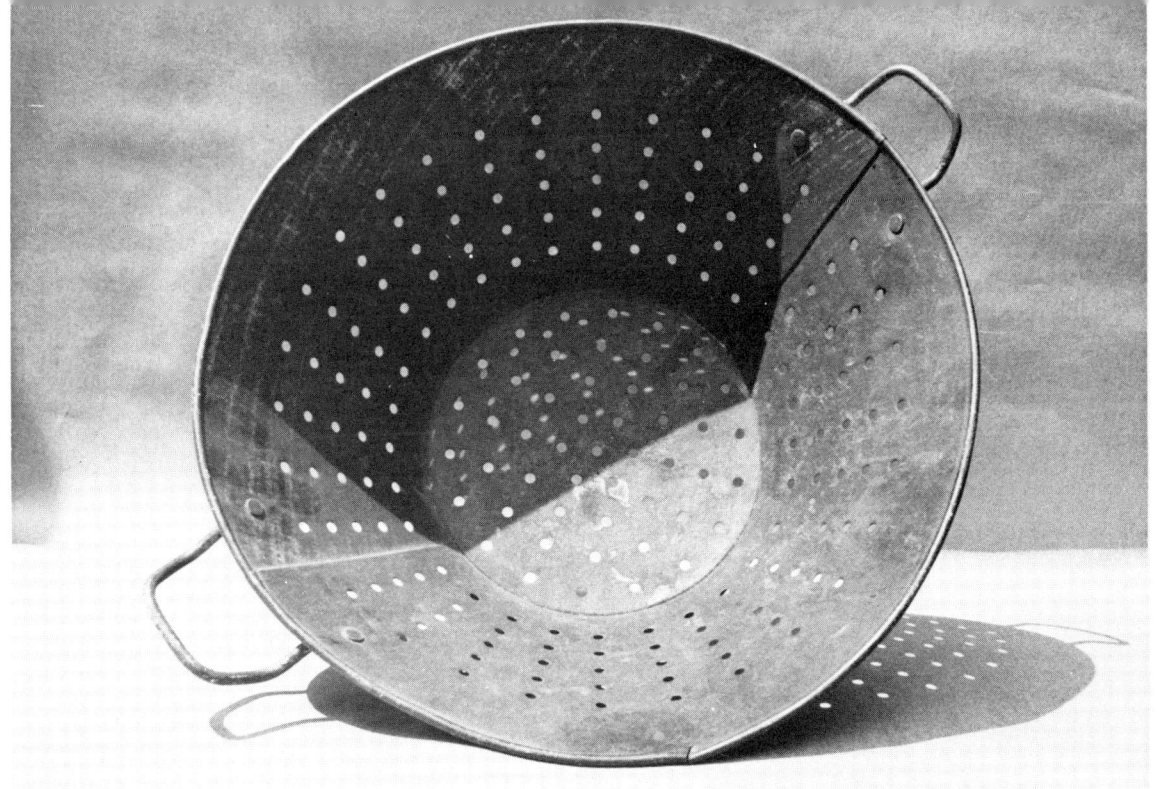

colander, then put them back in the water they were boiled in, together with four hard-boiled eggs quartered, and half a lemon sliced, a little pepper if you like it. Boil up and serve.

(*Allan's New England Almanack,* 1850)

This is almost a vegetable omelet. Serve it on toast for lunch or a light supper.

EGG BROCCOLI: Take half a dozen heads of broccoli, cut off the small shoots or blossoms and lay them aside for frying; trim the stalks short and pare off the rough rind up to the head; wash them well, and lay them in salt water for an hour; then put them in plenty of boiling water (salted) and let them boil fast till quite tender. Put two ounces of butter in a saucepan, and stir it over a slow fire till it is melted; then add gradually six or eight well beaten eggs, and stir the mixture until it is thick and smooth. Lay the broccoli in the centre of a large dish, pour the egg around it, and having fried the broccoli blossoms, arrange them in a circle near the edge of the dish.

(*Domestic Receipts,* 1860)

A delicious dish. Add a little grated Parmesan cheese to perk it up.

FRICASSED EGG PLANT: Having peeled and sliced the egg plants, boil them in water with a saltspoonful of salt, until they are thoroughly cooked. Drain off the water, pour in sufficient milk to cover the slices, and add a few bits of butter rolled in flour; let it simmer gently, shaking the pan over the fire till the sauce is thick, and stir in the beaten yolks of two or three eggs just before it is served.

(*Mrs. Winslow's Domestic Receipt Book,* 1868)

A superb side dish with charcoal broiled steak!

MRS. BADGER'S CORN GRIDDLES: To eat with meat—twelve ears sweet corn, grate off the grains, two eggs, pepper, salt and a very little butter, half teacup of flour, half teacup of milk, stir well together, and fry on a griddle.

(*Collected Receipts,* 1840)

This is also an excellent way to use up cold cooked leftover artichokes.

FRIED ARTICHOKES: Cut the artichokes into six or eight pieces, according to their size; remove the choke and the large leaves which will not become tender, and trim off the tops of the remaining leaves with a pair of scissors. Wash them in several waters, drain, and dip them in a batter made with flour, a little cream, and the yolk of egg. Let the artichokes be well covered with the batter, fry them in oil or in white dripping, sprinkle a little salt over them, and serve on a bed of parsley fried in the oil, &c., which remains in the pan.

(*Peterson's National Ladies Magazine,*
September 1860)

Egg & Cheese Dishes

I found this receipt for an omelet in an old handwritten cookbook without a date. Thomas Jefferson imported Parmesan cheese into the United States in the late 1700s, and it was in popular use by 1835, so this receipt dates somewhere in the mid-1800s. It also happens to be a very classical French method for making omelets, and you can use it as a basis for any number of fillings other than the suggested Parmesan cheese.

CHEESE OMELET: Beat up three eggs, with pepper and salt to taste, and two tablespoonfuls of grated Parmesan cheese. Put a piece of butter the size of an egg into the omelet-pan; as soon as it is melted, pour in the eggs, and, holding the handle of the pan with one hand, stir the omelet with the other by means of a flat spoon. The moment the omelet begins to set, cease stirring, but keep shaking the pan for a minute or so; then with the spoon double-up the omelet, and keep shaking the pan until the underside is of a good colour. Turn it out on a hot dish, coloured side upper-most, and serve quickly with Parmesan cheese sprinkled over it.

(old manuscript cookery book)

I don't think the next receipt needs much explanation as just about everyone is familiar with Welsh Rarebit, but familiar or not, this very simple receipt deserves to be tried at least once. It's much less complicated than most modern versions, and, to my taste, the results are as good or better.

WELSH RAREBIT: Take a large cupful of finely grated cheese; having seasoned to taste, add a well-beaten egg, and mix with new milk to the consistency of thick cream; put it into a pan, and when just boiling, pour over hot buttered toast. We have never had it either curdled or stringy by this method.

(*Peterson's National Ladies Magazine,* August 1866)

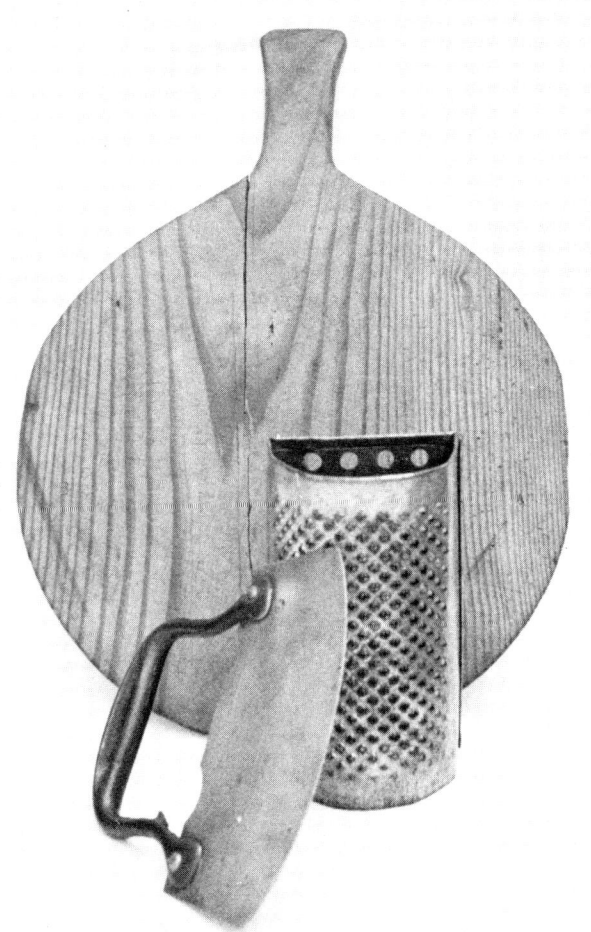

This dish is very nice done in those small soufflé dishes and served as a main course for lunch or a light supper. A good sharp Cheddar gives the best results.

A SAVOURY DISH: Melt a quarter-pound of good cheese in the oven. When sufficiently melted, add one egg and a wine-glass of milk. Beat together till it resembles a custard. Bake in a hot oven till light brown.

(*Household Receipts*, 1870)

Here's an omelet with a slightly crepe-like texture.

MRS. HOYLE'S OMELET: Four eggs well-beaten, as much milk as there is egg, and half tablespoon flour to each egg; a little salt and pepper; fry as you do any omelet.

(*Domestic Cookery*, 1855)

A great dish for Sunday brunch...

OUEFS DE LA CROQUEMITAINE: Put into a stewpan three tablespoonfuls of cream or milk, a little grated tongue or beef, pepper and salt. When quite hot, put in four eggs, well beaten; stir all the time until the mixture becomes quite thick. Have ready a slice of toasted bread well buttered; spread the mixture on the toast, and send it to table very hot.

(*Mrs. Winslow's Domestic Receipt Book*, 1870)

This custom was prevalent in the 1800s and seems to have disappeared at just about the turn of the century. Try it—it's one of those things you'll either love or hate.

EGG CREAM: Take the yolk of an egg with a dessert spoonful of cream or milk; this will serve for three people to mix with their tea. This is much used in Germany for invalids, and is both nourishing and palatable. The above has been recommended for disease of the lungs where there is difficulty breathing, short dry breath and cough, hectic towards evening, and night perspirations.

(*The Mother's Book Of Daily Duties*, 1855)

This sauce dresses up vegetables nicely, particularly asparagus and broccoli.

EGG SAUCE: Is made by putting two or three eggs, hardboiled, then minced fine, into melted butter. The butter need not be as thick when eggs are to be added.

(*Valuable Receipts*, 1830)

In case you were wondering why the previous receipt specifies "The butter need not be as thick when eggs are to be added," the following receipt should clear up any confusion.

MELTED BUTTER: Always use sweet butter; if in the least injured, it spoils the gravy. To make it of the best quality, cut two ounces of butter into little bits, put these in a clean stewpan, with a large teaspoonful of flour and a table-spoonful of milk. When thoroughly melted and mixed, add six table-spoonfuls of water, hold it over the fire, and shake it round every minute (all the time one way) till it just begins to simmer; then let it stand quietly and boil up. It should be of the thickness of good cream.

(*Valuable Receipts,* 1830)

Rich egg custards.

MILK CUSTARDS: Heat up a quart of milk quite hot, that it may not whey when baked; let it stand till cold; then mix with it eight eggs; sweeten with loaf sugar, and flavour with essence of lemon and rose water, or vanilla. Fill your cups, set them in an oven in a dripping pan half filled with boiling water. When the water has boiled ten or fifteen minutes take out a cup, and if the custard is of the consistency of jelly it is done. Cover the cups in the oven and they will bake better.

(*The American Domestic Cookbook,* 1868)

In case you've ever wanted to keep eggs for a while...

EGGS: These packed in salt or charcoal with the small end downward, well covered, will keep fresh two or three years.

(*Mrs. Winslow's Domestic Receipt Book,* 1868)

These used to be very popular as a snack. They're an especially good snack when you're on a diet—lots of protein and nourishment with few calories.

PICKLING EGGS: Prepare a spiced pickling liquid the same as for spiced cucumbers or other pickles. Or boil in a cloth bag for 15 or 20 minutes in 1 quart of white or pure cider vinegar, 1 ounce of raw ginger, 1 ounce of allspice, 2 blade of mace, 1 ounce of pepper, 1 ounce of salt, 3 or 4 cloves of garlic, and 1 ounce of mustard seed. Boil for this quantity of pickle, a dozen eggs for ten minutes. Place to cool in a pan of cold water. Remove the shells, pack them in a crock, and when perfectly cold, pour the pickling liquid over them. Lay over the top a folded cloth to keep the eggs under the pickling liquid, and tie over the top of the jar a thickness of cotton batting. They will be ready to use in about four weeks.

(*Household Discoveries,* 1871)

The carriage course leading to the house should be lined with locusts, cedar, ash, and other rare trees;—roses, and lilacs, and jasmine, and their sister beauties should be peeping through the boughs like so many fairies. We know God loves and cares for them, why should not we??

(*The Mother's Book Of Daily Duties,* 1855)

A man is like a good tree; the more full of fruits the branches are, the lower they bend.

(*Allan's New England Almanack,* 1792)

Desserts

A FEW GENERAL RULES
FOR CAKE MAKING & BAKING

One of my favorite old receipt books, *The Mother's Book Of Daily Duties Containing Hints and Directions For The Body, Mind And Character (Also A Brief And Comprehensive Guide For The Training Of Infants, Management Of Children, Nursing The Sick, Curing Diseases And Injuries; With Safe And Simple Remedies, And A Full List Of Miscellaneous Receipts For Family Use),* has a section on cakes and baking. Although many of the suggestions are no longer valid in the era of automatic ovens and pre-seeded raisins, most of the hints are helpful, or at the very least, entertaining!

A FEW GENERAL RULES FOR CAKE MAKING AND BAKING: A practical housekeeper learns by experience, that many little things are very important to success in the delicate art of making nice cake, and failures are often the result of seeming trifles. To obviate this, it is necessary to observe the following rules. If you want your cake white, use the white sugar, although the clear brown makes it equally good. For variety, it is well to make both.

In receipts where milk is used, it is not well to use a mixture of both sweet and sour, as it has a tendency to make the cake heavy.

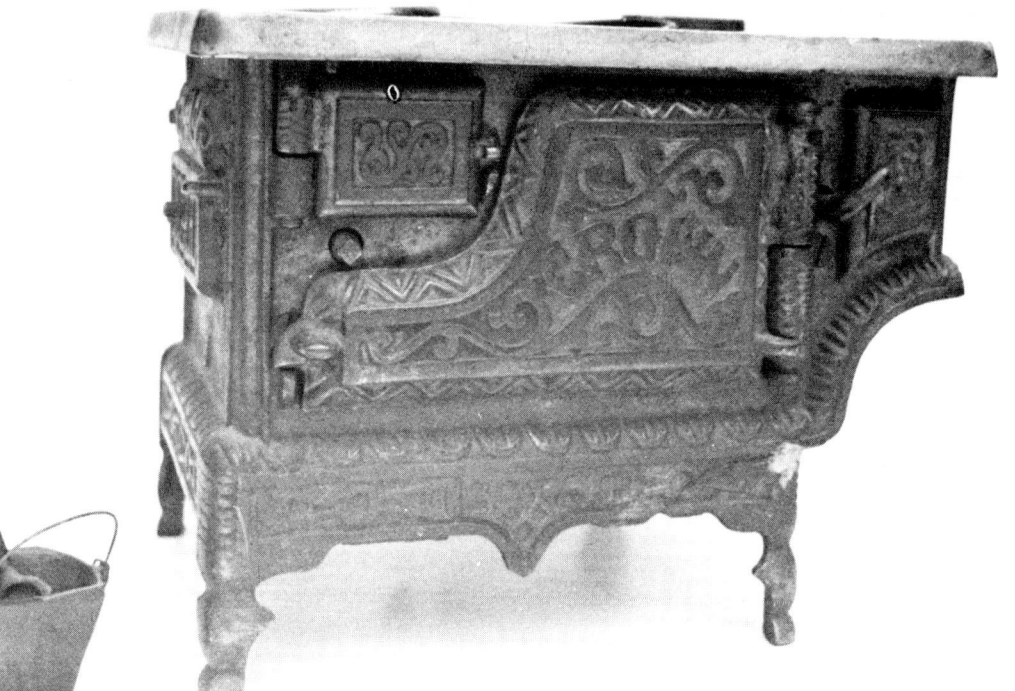

Butter used in a cake should be sweet, if rank or strong it will spoil it, the salt in the butter improves the taste if not too salt.

Roll the sugar fine, and beat the butter and sugar to a light cream, then beat the eggs till you can take up a spoonful. This is for common cake, but for sponge or other fine cake, follow the directions. When the parts are put together, the whole should be beat till light and creamy.

Before beginning, see that all your ingredients are before you, for by omitting a particle you may spoil your cake.

There is now in use a cheap article called the egg-beater, made of wire fastened into a handle, that requires far less time than any other mode, and makes a light froth in a few moments. It can be had for a shilling or eighteen pence, and is very easy to use. If you cannot obtain this, a whalebone split at the end in several parts is good. If you have neither, a fork will do.

A platter is best to beat the whites of eggs on, any dish will do for the cake, though earthen is thought to be best.

To blanch almonds, pour boiling water on them until the skins are easily removed, then throw them into cold water, to whiten them; drain them from the water to pound, but not wipe them dry, as the water prevents their oiling. Almonds should be pounded in a marble or hard wood mortar.

To ascertain when a cake is done, insert in the thickest part, a splint of a broom, and if no dough sticks, and it comes out clean, it is done. If the loaf is large, use a small knife blade in the same way.

For baking plum or other large cakes, use the round pans, those made with tubes in the center are best, as then the middle will bake as fast as the other parts. Pans with straight sides are the best. Line them with buttered white paper, and fill them not more than half full of batter. Long narrow deep tins are best for spongecakes, and should be prepared the same way. Much depends upon the baking; if this is not done right, you cannot have good cake; it is quite as often spoiled in the baking as in the making. The oven must have a regular heat through it, and particularly a good heat at the bottom, without which a cake will not rise. A *quick* oven is one in which you can only hold your hand in to count 25, a *slow* one, to count 30. Bread may go into an oven in which you can count but 20.

In using saleratus or sal volatile, it must be powdered, measured, and dissolved in a little warm water before putting to the cake, and should be the last thing added in all cookery.

A bit of volatile salts, and a piece of alum, each the size of a hickory nut, powdered fine and dissolved, added to sponge cake mixture, will insure a light cake. It is much used by cake bakers. It is generally put in with the beaten eggs, and beaten with them ten minutes or so.

Before making cake or bread, have your flour sifted and on the table, and your tins buttered. If your receipt is to be weighed, measure it after weighing, and note it down in your receipt book, and it will ever after save you the trouble.

Citron when used should be cut in thin strips; fresh orange or lemon peel should be grated before using, and raisins stoned and chopped and rubbed with flour. They will divide, and are not as likely to settle at the bottom. Fruitcake should be made a little thicker than other cake.

In making sponge cake, or any where the whites of the eggs are used separate, it requires *two* to beat both parts well. The whites should be whisked till they stand in a heap.

All cake without yeast should have the flour put in and then, when stirred, the saleratus just before baking.

Currants should be washed and dried for future use, and clean from stones.

If a cake bake too fast at first on the top and becomes hard, it will not be light. A paper should be laid over it before this is the case. If it burns at the bottom it injures the looks and the taste.

ICING FOR CAKES: For the whites of two eggs, take a quarter of a pound of powdered and sifted white sugar. The eggs should be beat to a high froth, and the sugar stirred in and flavoured with rose or lemon.

Another and easier rule is, to one egg ten large teaspoonful of sifted sugar prepared in the same way, beat till it will pile in a heap.

METHOD OF LAYING IT ON: If the sides are to be frosted, set the loaf on the bottom of the basin in which it was baked, and lay the icing over the sides with a broad bladed knife, then take another knife, dip it in water and smooth it over evenly; then ice the top, laying it on in a heap in the centre as much as will be needed, and then with a knife dipped in cold water, spread the icing evenly on the surface when the cake is cool. Set it in a warm place to dry. If the loaf is to be frosted all over, two whites are allowed, if only for the top, one will do. For two loaves three whites will answer.

Icing which is harder is made with the white of an egg, one teaspoonful of powdered sifted starch, and nine of sifted sugar, stirred ten or fifteen minutes together, prepared as the other; and two teaspoonsful of lemon juice, flavoured with rose water or lemon. Lay it on in twenty minutes of baking, and then set in a cool place to harden.

Frosting looks best, to be laid on twice—putting the first on soon after it comes from the oven, and the second the next day after the other is perfectly dry.

Ornamental frosting—for this purpose have a small syringe, draw it full of the icing and work it in any fancy design you fancy. Wheels, Grecian borders, grapes, or flowers look well, or borders of beading. It must not be put on till the plain frosting is cold and hard.

(*The Mother's Book Of Daily Duties,* 1855)

Cakes, Puddings, Pies & Preserves

Delicious:

APPLE FRITTERS: Make a batter with one cup of milk, one teaspoonful of sugar, two eggs, whites and yolks beaten separately, two cups of flour, one teaspoonful of baking powder mixed with the flour. Chop up a few good tart apples, mix in the batter, and fry in hot lard. They are delicious if served with maple syrup.

(*McCall's,* December 1875)

This receipt will probably baffle anyone who isn't a seasoned baker, but for those of you who are familiar with yeast doughs it's a very interesting cake to make—the texture is very much like modern-day babka.

A FRENCH CAKE: Out of two pounds of flour take one-half pound, make a hole in the centre, and put in one-quarter ounce of yeast, mixed with a little warm but not hot water; make it into a sponge, and place it, well-wrapped up, in a warm place. When the leaven has risen sufficiently, which will be known by its having increased in bulk by half, make a hole in the centre of the remaining flour, and put in one pound of butter and six eggs; work it well-together, so as to make a soft sponge, which must be kneaded twice with the hands; if too stiff, another egg must be added. Cut up and stone a quarter-pound of Malaga raisins, add the same quantity of dried currants and some sugar, mix all the ingredients well-together with the sponge; add the leaven, put it into a well-buttered tin mold, and let the whole stand for an hour or two to rise. When well-risen, bake in a moderate oven for an hour or an hour and a quarter.

(*Peterson's National Ladies Magazine,* July 1871)

I have several friends who fancy themselves connoisseurs of rice pudding, and the following receipt is their all-time favorite.

HUNTINGTON PUDDING: One pint of milk and half a teacupful of rice, put into a tin and set in a pot nearly halfful of boiling water; keep the water boiling until the rice is steamed soft enough to yield when pressed with the thumb and finger; then add the yolks of two eggs, a small lump of butter, eating raisins to taste, and the grated rind of lemon; turn into a pudding dish, beat the whites to a stiff froth, and stir in three ounces of sugar and the juices of a lemon; spread the frosting on the pudding, and put into the oven to brown.

(*Household Receipts,* 1865)

This cake is said to have been Dolly Madison's favorite. For the saleratus, substitute one tablespoonful of baking powder and a teaspoonful of baking soda. This cake is one of my favorites because it is very much like a Christmas fruitcake without all the candied citron and nuts.

MRS. MADISON'S WHIM: Two pounds of flour, two pounds of sugar, two pounds of butter beaten into a cream, twelve eggs, the yolks beaten with the sugar and the whites to a high froth, half a teacupful of rosewater, or lemon brandy in which the rinds have been soaked, two nutmegs grated, and one teaspoonful of saleratus dissolved. Beat all together well, then add two pounds of raisins stoned and chopped. Bake in a quick oven. This cake is good for three month's keeping.

(*Mrs. Foster's Receipts,* 1845)

These "cakes" are really cookies and are a perfect accompaniment to after-dinner coffee.

> LEMON DROP CAKE: Grate the rinds from three large lemons, put it to three heaping tablespoonsful of white powdered sugar, and a tablespoonful of flour; work the whole well together with the white of one egg. Drop in small cakes on buttered paper about an inch apart. Bake in a slow oven.
>
> (*Mrs. Foster's Receipts,* 1845)

Blanc Mange is still a part of our cuisine, but I've found this receipt to make a slightly different version, particularly if you use ground rice as the thickening agent. If you don't have any molds you can simply pour it into small dessert dishes. I usually serve these with sliced fresh fruit (strawberries, peaches, etc.) and custard sauce. The best part is that they may be made a day or two ahead.

> BLANC MANGE PUDDING: One quart of milk scalded, six tablespoonful of ground rice washed—wheat flour may be used for this—, stirred in smoothly, a piece of butter the size of a walnut, the whole stirred into the milk, and boiling it fifteen minutes, stirring it constantly. Remove it from the fire, and stir in a quarter of a teaspoonful of extract of lemon, and the same of dry soda, and let it stand ten minutes. Wet the molds in cold water, and fill them, to cool. When perfectly cold, turn on a platter, preserving the shape neatly, and serve with a soft custard and raspberry jam.
>
> (*The Mother's Book Of Daily Duties,* 1850)

A really delicious rich dessert!

> GENOESE CREAM: One pint of milk boiled, the yolks of three eggs beaten, one heaping spoonful of flour, two of sugar, stirred in a little cold milk, and a piece of butter half the size of an egg, the batter stirred into the hot milk, and boiled ten minutes. Stir in the eggs, and then turn out. Flavour with lemon, or anything you please. Blanch half a pound of almonds, and chop them fine, and stir in one half into the cream. Dip slices of sponge cake in sweet wine, and lay around the dish, and pour the cream over the cake, and lay the rest of the almonds over the whole. A nice dessert for dinner, or parties, or a New Year's table.
>
> (Mrs. L. G. Abell, 1855)

Another cake named after a famous personality of the day.

> HENRY CLAY CAKE: One pound of flour and one pound of sugar, one ounce of butter, half a pint of cream; one teaspoonful of soda, one lemon, and half a nutmeg. Bake well in a medium oven.
>
> (*Mrs. Foster's Receipts,* 1850)

I use pound cake in place of the toast and serve it with whipped cream.

PLUMB CHARLOTTE: Stone a quart of ripe Plumbs and stew them with three quarters of a pound of brown sugar. Cut thin slices of bread and butter it, lay it in the sides and on the bottom of the dish, pour in your Plumbs boiling hot and cover again with bread and butter, put in a cold place and when perfectly cold, turn it out on a flat dish. Eat with cream and sugar.

(*The Mother's Book Of Daily Duties,* 1850)

After adding the chocolate taste to see if it's chocolaty enough—I generally double the amount. For those of you accustomed to commercial chocolate pudding this is bound to be a real treat.

CHOCOLATE PUDDING: One quart of sweet milk, three ounces of grated chocolate. Scald the milk and chocolate together; when cool, add the yolks of five eggs and one cup of sugar. Bake about twenty-five minutes; beat the whites for the top, brown in the oven; eat cold.

(*Mrs. Winslow's Domestic Receipt Book,* 1870)

An apple-flavored cake—spicy and different.

CIDER CAKE #2: Four and one-half cups flour, one and two-thirds cups sugar, one teaspoon soda, three-fourths cup butter, one and one-third cider, one teaspoon cinnamon, two-thirds teaspoon cloves. Bake in a medium oven till done.

(*Mrs. Winslow's Domestic Receipt Book,* 1870)

No collection of colonial cakes would be complete without at least one good old-fashioned gingerbread.

AUGUSTA'S MOLASSES GINGERBREAD: One egg, one tablespoon butter, two-thirds cup molasses, half cup milk, one teaspoon soda, two and one-half cups flour, one tablespoon ginger, one teaspoon cream of tartar, salt; sour milk may be used, but if so, use one cup, two teaspoons soda, and no cream of tartar. Bake in a hot oven.

(*Mrs. Winslow's Domestic Receipt Book,* 1870)

With regard to sin, fear is the greatest bravery.

(*Beer's Almanac,* 1834)

No one bothers to make their own anymore, but if you're willing to try these once, you may never buy crackers again.

CRACKERS: One pint water, one teacup butter, one teaspoonful soda, two of cream tartar, flour enough to make as stiff as biscuit. Let them stand in the oven till dried through. They do not need pounding.

(*The Mother's Book Of Daily Duties,* 1850)

Another colonial standby was cornbread. Use baking soda for the saleratus.

INDIAN MEAL BREAKFAST CAKES: Pour boiling water into a quart of yellow corn-meal; stir it until wet; then add two well-beaten eggs, and milk enough to make a thick batter; measure a small teaspoonful of dry saleratus, and dissolve it in warm water, and put it to the batter with the same quantity of salt; butter square tin pans, fill them two-thirds full, and bake in a quick oven for one hour; when done, cut it in small squares, and serve hot.

(*Dr. Herrick's American Domestic Receipt Book,* 1868)

Cakes of this type must have been a big treat in colonial days; I can't imagine too many wives who had the time to beat a cake for an *hour!* I make this cake without the caraway seeds and beat it for half an hour (with an electric mixer). If you like a good old-time pound cake, you've got to try this.

POUND SEED CAKE: One pound of butter beaten to a cream, one pound of sifted lump sugar, one pound of flour well-dried, eight eggs, yolks and whites beaten separately, and caraway seeds to taste. Mix the ingredients, and beat all well-together for one hour. Put the batter into a tin shape, well-lined with paper and buttered. Bake in a moderate oven.

(*Mrs. Abell's Receipts,* 1860)

A nice variation on sugar cookies...

SWEET BISCUITS: Rub four ounces of butter into eight ounces of flour, add six ounces of ground loaf sugar, the yolks of two eggs, the white of one, add a tablespoonful of brandy; roll the paste thin, and cut it with a wine-glass or cutter; egg over the tops of each with the remaining white, and sift on sugar; bake in a moderate oven.

(*Mrs. Foster's Receipts,* 1845)

A simple white cake to which you may add a tablespoonful of brandy or vanilla extract.

PLAIN CAKE: Take three-quarters of a pound of flour, one-quarter pound of currants, two teaspoonfuls of baking powder, one egg, and nearly half a pint of milk. The powder to be mixed with the flour and milk when going into the oven.

(*The Mother's Book Of Daily Duties,* 1855)

Basically an English muffin. I use tuna fish cans with both ends cut out for the hoops (place them on a cookie sheet before you put in the batter), and two packages of dry yeast.

TEA CAKES: Two pounds of flour, one and a-half pints of warm milk, in which two and a-half ounces of butter are to be melted, and a large tablespoonful of yeast. Mix well-together, and beat up sharply for some time; then put the mixture into tin hoops, from two and a-half inches to three inches deep (which should be buttered inside) and leave them near the fire to rise for a little while before you put them in the oven. Do not fill the hoops more than half-full with the mixture.

(*Helpful Receipts,* 1850)

I've been enjoying this since I was able to eat solid food, and I still think it's one of the nicest desserts imaginable. This receipt was handwritten by my great-grandmother about 1850.

THE QUEEN OF PUDDINGS: One pint of breadcrumbs, one quart of milk, six ounces of sugar, butter the size of an egg, the yolks of four eggs. Flavor with lemon, and bake as a custard. Beat the whites of the four eggs to a stiff froth, mix with a cup of powdered sugar and the juice of a lemon. Spread a layer of fruit-jelly over the custard while hot; cover with the frosting, and bake until slightly brown. To be eaten cold with cream, or warm with any sauce that may be preferred.

If you like to make your tapioca pudding with regular tapioca rather than the instant variety, this receipt is one of the best I've found.

TAPIOCA PUDDING: Put three tablespoonfuls of tapioca to soak over night in lukewarm water; in the morning, pour on this one quart of milk; and set it on the stove till it comes to a boil; add a pinch of salt, and four or five tablespoonfuls of white sugar, the yolks of three eggs, which, when you pour in, cools it; let it come to a boil again, or until it thickens, stirring all the time; then pour in

Envy deserves more pity than anger. It makes the one who feels it, extremely unhappy. Whoever envies another, *admits their superiority.*
(*The Family Almanack,* 1838)

your pudding dish; then beat the whites of the three eggs to a froth, add four tablespoonfuls of powdered sugar, and spread over the tapioca; put it in the oven, and bake a light brown.

(*The Mother's Book Of Daily Duties,* 1855)

Just in case you ever have a reason to make rice pudding without eggs...

RICE PUDDING WITHOUT EGGS: Put into a well-buttered dish a quarter-pound of the best Carolina rice simply washed, pour on it three pints of cold milk, sweeten and flavour to taste; put a little butter and nutmeg on the top to brown; bake two hours and a-half in a slow oven, on which much of the success of the pudding depends.

(*Peterson's National Ladies Magazine,* 1868)

You can make this with prepared applesauce; use chunky-style if possible.

APPLE SNOW: Stew two pounds of apples with four ounces of loaf sugar until tender. Beat the yolks of six eggs with two ounces of loaf sugar, and pour over them one pint of boiling milk. Put this custard into a kettle, and cook until it is as thick as corn-flour pudding. Beat the whites of six eggs to a stiff froth, with one tablespoon powdered sugar. Put the apples in a dish, pour custard over them, cover this with the frosting, place in the oven, and brown lightly.

(*Mrs. Smyth's Household Receipts,* 1855)

Here's a receipt that resembles Apple Snow. You can also use apple sauce in this version, which will considerably cut down the time needed to make it.

APPLE TRIFLE (A SUPPER DISH): Ten good-sized apples, the rind of half a lemon, six ounces of pounded sugar, half a pint of milk, half a pint of cream, whipped, two eggs. Peel, core, and cut the apples into thin slices, and put them into a saucepan with two tablespoonfuls of water, the sugar, and minced lemon-rind. Boil all together until quite tender, and pulp the apples through a sieve; if they should not be quite sweet enough, add a little more sugar, and put them at the bottom of the dish to form a thick layer. Stir together the milk, cream, and eggs, with a little sugar, over the fire, and let the mixture thicken, but do not allow it to reach the boiling point. When thick, take off the fire; let it cool a little, then pour it over the apples. Whip some cream with sugar, lemon juice, etc., the same as for other trifles; heap it high over the custard, and the dish is ready for the table. It may be garnished, as fancy dictates, with strips of bright apple jelly, slices of citron, etc.

(Mrs. Winslow's Domestic Receipt Book, 1870)

This is delectable made with acorn or butternut squash.

SQUASH PIE: Pare, take out the seeds, and stew the squash till very soft and dry. Strain or rub it through a sieve or collander. Mix this with good milk or cream till it is thick as batter; sweeten it with sugar. Allow five eggs to a quart of milk, beat the eggs well, add them to the squash, and season with rose-water, cinnamon, nutmeg, or whatever spices you like. Line a pie-plate with crust, fill and bake about an hour.

(Valuable Receipts, 1860)

A good old-fashioned receipt for good old-fashioned pumpkin pie.

PUMPKIN PIE: Stew the pumpkin dry, and make it like squash pie, only season rather higher. In the country, where this real yankee pie is prepared in perfection, ginger is almost always used with the other spices. There, too, cream instead of milk is mixed with the pumpkin, which gives it a richer flavour. Roll the paste rather thicker than for fruit pies, as there is but one crust. If the pie is large and deep, it will require an hour to bake in a brisk oven.

(Valuable Receipts, 1860)

Each housewife used to have her own special receipt for mincemeat. This is a very basic version which you may vary to taste.

FAMILY MINCE PIES: Boil three pounds of lean beef till tender, and when cold chop it fine. Chop three pounds of clear beef suet, and mix the meat, sprinkling in a table-spoonful of salt. Pare, core, and chop fine six pounds of good apples; stone four pounds of raisins, and chop them; wash and dry two pounds of currants; and mix them well with the meat. Season with a spoonful of powdered cinnamon, a powdered nutmeg, a little mace, and a few cloves, pounded, and one pound of brown sugar; add a quart of Madeira wine and half a pound of citron cut into small bits. This mixture put in a stone jar and closely covered will keep several weeks. It makes a rich pie for Thanksgiving and Christmas.

(Mrs. Foster's Receipts, 1845)

A very unusual lemon pie.

LEMON PIE: For one pie, take a couple of good-sized fresh lemons, squeeze out the juice, and mix it with half a pint of molasses, or sufficient sugar to make the juice sweet. Chop the peel fine, line a deep pie-plate with your pastry, then sprinkle on a layer of your chopped lemon peel, turn in part of the mixed sugar and molasses and juice, then cover the whole with pie crust, rolled very thin.— Put in another layer of peel, sweetened juice, and crust, and so, till all the lemon is used. Cover the whole with a thick crust, and bake the pie about half an hour.

(*The Married Ladies Companion,* 1850)

If you can get hold of some quinces and good green cooking apples, this is an interesting pie to make. I slice the apples, and season with a bit of nutmeg and cinnamon, with a sprinkling of lemon juice. Any good pie crust may be used.

TO MAKE A PYE WITH PIPPINS: Pare your pippins, and cut out the cores, then make your coffin of crust. Take a good handful of quinces sliced and lay at the bottom, then lay your pippins on top, and fill the holes where the core was taken out with sirup of quinces, then pour on the top the sirup of quinces, then put in sugar, and close it up, let it be very well baked, for it will ask much soaking, especially the quinces.

(*The Compleat Cook's Guide,* 1683)

Apple Pandowdy was standard breakfast fare in the fall, though today it is preferred as a dinner dessert. Instead of baking all night, the following revisions make for better results: in a 350° oven bake the apples until they are soft, then cover with a rich baking powder biscuit and bake for fifteen or twenty minutes longer.

APPLE PANDOWDY: Using a deep dish of earthenware or iron, take five or six sliced apples, 3 table-spoons sugar, 4 table-spoons molasses, nutmeg, cinnamon, and salt to taste, and mix all together in the dish. Cover with a baking powder biscuit crust extending over the sides. Bake overnight. In the morning cut the hard crust into the apple. Eat with yellow cream or plain.

(*Receipts in Cookery,* 1879)

The colonials' methods of preserving food were limited by the equipment available at the time. Nowadays we have at our disposal canning jars and methods that are much more reliable, not to mention safer. The following receipts for pickles, relishes, jams and preserves should be sealed, using the water-bath method. If you're

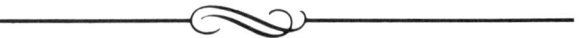

The real merit of a man should be estimated by his virtue, not by his fortune.

(*Strong's Astrological Diary,* 1800)

familiar with canning and preserving this will be a procedure you've already mastered, but, if not, I suggest you send for the "Ball Blue Book" which details all the various methods and which will give you all the information you need to can successfully. It is available for 50¢ from The Ball Corporation; Muncie, Indiana 47302.

The following advice is as valid today as it was in 1865...

PRESERVING DAY: Many housekeepers prefer, when putting up fruits for home use, to preserve a jar or two each day, selecting the finest fruits as they ripen. Thus the labour is distributed over the entire season and associated with other cooking from day to day so as to be hardly realized. But it is of some advantage, when a considerable quantity of fruit is to be preserved, to get everything in readiness at one time and make a day of it.

(*The American Domestic Receipt Book,* 1865)

Almost as all-American as apple pie....

APPLE PRESERVES: Pippins are considered among the best apples for preserves. They may be cut in quarters. Weigh, and to each pound allow a pound of granulated sugar and a half pint of boiling water. Place the sugar and water upon the stove and let it come to a boil. Continue to boil vigorously for about twenty to thirty minutes. Place the apples in the boiling syrup and allow them to simmer until about half done. Then grate the rind of 1 and the juice of 2 lemons into this, and allow the whole to cook slowly until it is possible to run a straw through each of the quarters. When done, place in jars as before mentioned. [Place in jars, seal, and process in a boiling water bath for 20 minutes.] Some people preserve apples in brass or copper kettles. Others prefer bright new tins. But porcelain or graniteware are preferable to either. Never, in any case, use an old half-worn tin, as both the sirup and preserves will have a much clearer appearance if cooked in new tin or porcelain.

(*Houschold Receipts,* 1870)

Here's another apple receipt that was very popular.

APPLE MARMALADE: Take any kind of sour apples, pare and core them, cut them in small pieces, and to every pound of apples put three-fourths of a pound of sugar. Put them in a preserving pan and boil over a slow fire until they are reduced to a fine pulp. Then put in jelly jars, and keep them in a cool place. [Seal with parafin.]

(*Mrs. Winslow's Domestic Receipt Book,* 1871)

Apricot preserves are undoubtedly one of the most delicious breakfast treats ever created, and they're so easy to make!

APRICOT PRESERVES: Pare the fruit very thin and stone it. Use sugar, pound for pound, with the fruit. Place in a porcelain, graniteware, or earthenware vessel a layer of fruit to a layer of sugar, and let stand for a day. Next day boil very gently until they are clear. Remove them into a bowl and pour the liquor over them. The following day pour the liquor into a quart of codlin liquor. This is made by boiling and straining a pound of fine sugar with just enough water to make a sirup. Let the whole boil quickly until it will jelly. Put the fruit in and bring it to a boil, being careful to remove all scum. Then put up in small jars. [Place in jars, seal with parafin.]

(*Success Magazine*, 1889)

Preserved ginger isn't as popular today as it was a hundred years ago, but it's so good there's no reason why you shouldn't start your own revival.

TO PRESERVE GINGER: There is no better confection, perhaps, if properly made than preserved ginger. The young roots should be scalded until they become tender. Then peel them in cold water, changing the water frequently. Make a thin sirup, pour over the ginger roots, and let them stand for five days. Then remove them to the jars and pour over the ginger a rich sirup highly spiced. The sirup should be hot when it is poured over the ginger. [Place in jars, seal, and process in a boiling water bath for 15 minutes.]

(*Household Receipts*, 1852)

If you enjoy the flavor of molasses, this receipt is bound to be one of your favorites.

PEARS PRESERVED IN MOLASSES: Use hard pears. Cut the blossom ends, leaving on the stem. Peel, drop in cold water and put on the fire. Heat gradually and stew until tender. Remove the pears from the liquid and place in a dish where they can be kept warm at the side of the range. To each pound of liquid in which the fruit was cooked add a pint of molasses. Return to the fire, add a little ginger, and boil for half an hour. Take off the scum as it rises. Again place the pears in the liquid and cook for twenty minutes. They should be packed very tightly in jars and sealed while hot. [Place in jars, seal, and process in a boiling water bath for 20 minutes.]

(*Preserving Fruit*, 1870)

These are delicious served cold with whipped cream.

GINGER PEARS: Peel ripe pears, remove the cores, and cut into thin slices. To 4 pounds of pears allow the juice of 2 large lemons, 3½ pounds of sugar, and ¼ pound of ginger root scraped and cut into thin slices. To this add about a gill of water. Mix all together, except the lemon juice and the fruit. Place over the fire and heat until the sugar is dissolved. Then drop in the pears, add the lemon juice, and boil slowly for one hour. Can while hot. [Place in jars, seal, and process in a boiling water bath for 20 minutes.]

(*Peterson's National Ladies Magazine*, 1881)

A jar of this lemon flavoring is great to have on hand, and it keeps fine in a covered jar in the refrigerator.

TO PRESERVE LEMON PEEL: Make a thick syrup of white sugar, chop the lemon peel fine, and boil in the syrup ten minutes. Put in glass tumblers and paste paper over them. A teaspoonful of this may be used to improve a loaf cake or dish of sauce.

(*The Ladies Companion*, 1873)

Easy, but when you taste this jelly you'll never believe you could end up with such good results for so little effort.

CRANBERRY JELLY: To one quart of cranberries put a quart of water, and boil them to a pulp; mash them with a wooden ladle whilst boiling; then strain them; and, to each pint of the juice, add a half pound of loaf-sugar; set it over a slow fire, and stir with a silver spoon; try it often, by taking some of it into a saucer. When cold, if it is not a fine jelly, continue to boil until it is so. [Place in jars, seal, and process in a boiling water bath for 20 minutes.]

(*Dr. Herrick's American Domestic Receipt Book*, 1868)

This fruit jam receipt may be used for just about any fruit. Little has been done to improve it in two hundred years.

RASPBERRY JAM: To each pound of fruit allow three-quarters of a pound of white sugar. Mash the berries, mix all together, boil, stir, and skim. The jam will be done in half an hour. Put into warm glasses, and seal up, or tie papers on the top. Other jams are made in the same way. [Place in jars and seal with parafin.]

(*The Mother's Book Of Daily Duties*, 1850)

This receipt makes a delicious pineapple preserve which is very crisp and unusual because it isn't cooked. I find the easiest way to store these is in the refrigerator.

PINE APPLES PRESERVED WITHOUT COOKING: Pare and shave them very thin; to a pound of the fruit, use a pound and a half of double refined sugar. Lay a layer of sugar in a stone jar, and then one of the fruit, till all is packed. The next day stir them up with a wooden spoon, and repeat it, once or twice a day, for three days. Then put them in glass jars, seal them tight, and pack them in salt, and thus they will keep for years, and are as clear as honey, and perfectly delicious in flavour.

(*The Mother's Book Of Daily Duties,* 1850)

This is a good way to use up two or three extra pears and make a very nice dessert. They'll keep refrigerated in a well-sealed jar for about a month. With a scoop of vanilla ice cream they make a super last minute dessert.

PEARS WHOLE: Take the Vergaloo, or some other fine pears, leave the stem on, and pare them neatly. Take half a pound of sugar to a pound of fruit. Take a part of the sugar, and add sufficient water to boil them tender. Use a kettle large at the bottom, and only cook at once what will just cover it. When tender, add enough sugar to form a syrup, and when boiled half an hour, take them out, and do the remainder in the same manner, till finished. They will look, and are, very fine.

(*Mrs. Abell's Receipts,* 1850)

This is a relish that used to be found in every pantry, and it's a shame it isn't as common today because it's really good!

PICKLED PEACHES: Take ripe, sound clingstone peaches; remove the down with a brush; to a gallon of good vinegar made hot, add four pounds of coarse brown sugar; boil it down and skim it clear; stick five or six cloves in each peach, put them into a stone jar, and strain the vinegar over them whilst hot, cover the vessel and set it in a cold place for a few days, then drain off the vinegar, make it boiling hot again, strain it over, and set them away. Freestone peaches may be used.

(*Dr. Herrick's American Domestic Receipt Book,* 1868)

You'll never appreciate what "old-fashioned goodness" means until you try some homemade catsup.

TOMATO CATSUP: Wash the tomatoes, cut them in pieces, heat them soft, put through a cullender, then through a sieve. To a gallon of the juice, put four tablespoonfuls of salt, four of black pepper, three of mustard, one half tablespoonful of cloves, one teaspoonful cayenne pepper, one quart onions (cut up very fine), one pint of vinegar; simmer over a slow fire three or four hours, cork tight and keep in a cool cellar.

(*Dr. Herrick's American Domestic Receipt Book,* 1865)

Yet another way to prepare blackberries. You'll find this is a great accompaniment to cold meats and a great trick for making leftover meat seem like some exotic creation!

MARY'S PICKLED BLACKBERRIES: Three quarts blackberries, one quart vinegar, one quart sugar. No spice is required; put all together at the same time into your kettle and boil ten or fifteen minutes. After standing a few weeks they are very nice.

(*Mrs. Winslow's Domestic Receipt Book,* 1871)

This spiced fruit relish is wonderful to have on hand for perking up an otherwise bland meal.

ANNIE'S SPICED CURRANTS: Four quarts ripe currants, three and one-half pounds brown sugar, one pint of vinegar, one tablespoonful allspice, one tablespoonful cloves, and a little nutmeg. Boil one hour, stirring occasionally.

(*Mrs. Winslow's Domestic Receipt Book,* 1870)

Here's a simple, delicious way to use up extra apples and make a delicious dessert at the same time. You can also add a stick of cinnamon in the center of each apple.

A NICE WAY TO PREPARE APPLES: Pare a dozen, or as many as you desire, tart apples, take out the core, place sugar, with a small lump of butter in the centre of each apple, put them in a pan with a half pint of water, bake until tender, basting occasionally with the syrup while baking; when done, serve with cream.

(*Domestic Cookery,* 1840)

A superb relish, and don't let the quantities scare you off—just halve or quarter the amounts.

TIB'S GREEN TOMATO PICKLE: Slice one peck green tomatoes, six green peppers and four onions, and chop them. Strew one cup salt

A man who kept a tipling house, asked his neighbor what he should put upon his sign.—Write, said the neighbor, "Beggars made here!"
(*Beer's Almanac,* 1806)

over them in layers; let them stand one night. The next day turn the water off them, and put them in a kettle with a cup of grated horseradish, one tablespoon ground cloves, same of allspice and cinnamon. Cover with vinegar; boil soft, cover tight. Ready to eat in three days.

(Mrs. Winslow's Domestic Receipt Book, 1871)

Perhaps one of the greatest—and easiest to make—gourmet fruit treats.

BRANDY PEACHES: Drop the peaches in hot water, let them remain till the skin can be ripped off; make a thin syrup, and let it cover the fruit; boil the fruit till they can be pierced with a straw; take it out, make a very rich syrup, and add, after it is taken from the fire, and while it is still hot, an equal quantity of brandy. Pour this, while it is still warm, over the peaches in the jar. They must be covered with it.

(Dr. Herrick's American Domestic Receipt Book, 1865)

This is the only receipt I've ever run across for pumpkin marmalade. It's really good and *very* different! Just the thing to make out of those leftover decorative pumpkins the day after Halloween.

PUMPKIN MARMALADE: Take ripe, yellow pumpkins, pare and cut them in large pieces, scraping out the seeds with an iron spoon. Weigh the pieces, and to every pound allow one pound of the best double-refined sugar, and a small orange or lemon. Grate the piece of pumpkin on a coarse grater; powder the sugar and put it into a preserving kettle with grated pumpkin, the yellow rind of the orange grated, and the juice strained. Let all boil slowly, stirring it frequently, and skimming it well, till all is smooth, thick marmalade; put it warm into small glass jars or tumblers, lay a double round of tissue paper with a bladder or waxed paper. [Place in jars, seal, and process in a boiling water bath for 20 minutes.]

(Mrs. Winslow's Domestic Receipt Book, 1860)

One of the simplest and best-tasting cucumber pickle receipts I've ever made, and it works just fine with grocery store cukes....

MRS. NYE'S RIPE CUCUMBER PICKLES: Six pounds seed cucumbers—take out the seeds and cut in strips—one pound brown sugar, one tablespoon each cloves, allspice, cinnamon, pepper, two tablespoons salt; cover with vinegar and boil till tender.

(Mrs. Foster's Receipts, 1845)

I buy a bushel of apples in the fall and dry all of them using the following receipt. A "slack oven" used to mean an oven after the fire was out. To approximate this, preheat your oven to about 250° and then turn it off before putting the apples in.

PRESSED APPLES: Choose some firm, sound apples, not too ripe, (those called Stone Pippins are the best); put them on a baking dish in a slack oven, and leave them all night. In the morning take them out and pinch them, one at a time, between your finger and thumb, working all around each. Put them into the oven again at night, and pinch them in the morning, and continue doing both until they are soft enough. Then place them between two boards, with a weight upon them, so as to press them flat, but not so heavy as to burst them, and let them dry slowly.

(*Dr. Herrick's American Domestic Cook Book,* 1868)

Here's a nice version of apple jelly that's easy to make. Add a few drops of essence of peppermint and you'll have a very flavorful mint jelly to serve with lamb.

APPLE JELLY: Take any quantity of green juicy apples, peel them, cut them in four, and put them in cold water; put them in a brass pan, cover them with water (cold), put in a piece of white ginger, cover them, and let them boil until they are soft; pour them into a flannel bag, and let it run till you have as much juice as you require. Allow a pound of lump sugar for every pint of juice, clarify, and boil the sugar candy height, put in the juice, and boil for ten minutes; take a little drop in a saucer, set it to cool; if jellied, it is done; if not, boil a little longer, and add a few drops of essence of lemon.

(*Peterson's National Ladies Magazine,* 1871)

If you're fortunate enough to have a quince bush or are able to find them at your greengrocer's, do try this receipt. Quinces are a real taste treat. They're of no use raw, but either preserved or made into jelly the flavor is absolutely sublime.

PRESERVED QUINCES: Pare, quarter, and core the fruit, saving the skins and cores. Put the quinces over the fire with just enough water to cover them, and simmer until perfectly tender, but do not

A country jeweler advertises that he has a number of precious stones to dispose of—adding that "they sparkle like the tears of a young widow."

(Isaiah Thomas, *Junr's Almanac,* 1809)

let them break. Take out the fruit, and spread on dishes to cool; add the parings and cores to the water in which the quinces were boiled, and cook one hour; then strain through a jelly-bag, and to each pint of this liquor allow one pound of sugar. Boil and skim this; then put in the fruit, and boil again fifteen minutes. Take out the fruit, and spread on dishes to cool; boil down the syrup thick; put the fruit in your jars until two-thirds full, then cover with the syrup.

(*Peterson's National Ladies Magazine,* July 1881)

The colonials' favorite fruit could easily have been rhubarb, though today this wonderful dessert is no longer popular. Next time you see a bunch for sale, buy it and try it at least once. You won't be disappointed.

RHUBARB: To one pound of rhubarb, cut in pieces of one or two inches in length, allow one-half pound of loaf sugar, and the grated rind of one lemon. Have ready a large tin saucepan of boiling water, throw the rhubarb in, and stir the pieces down with a silver spoon—not one of iron or pewter. Put the cover on, and for three or four minutes it may be left, then the cover taken off; the rhubarb is not again left until done. It may be quietly turned in the saucepan with the spoon so as not to break the rhubarb. The moment it boils, it softens, and in three minutes or less time, according to whether the rhubarb is old or young. Strain it off quickly with the cover tilted on the saucepan, as in straining potatoes, leaving about a pint of water in to serve it with. Gently let it slip from the saucepan into a pie-dish; now as gently scatter the loaf-sugar and the grated lemon-rind over it, and leave until cold. The rhubarb should not be broken. A quarter of an hour is sufficient for this process of cooking rhubarb. The juice as well as the rind of the lemon may be used, if desired.

(*The Mother's Book Of Daily Duties,* 1855)

Toilet & Beauty Preparations

"A perfectly safe and innocent employment"

From the beginning of time women have been using all sorts of cosmetics and beauty treatments in an attempt to make themselves more beautiful and desirable. Colonial women were no exception, and many of the cosmetics they made and used are as effective today as they were then. The women who created these receipts used what was available, and this is what makes these preparations so valid today: They are made with wholesome and unadulterated ingredients.

The recent trend in "natural" and "organic" cosmetics is very sensible, but the problem is that most of the so-called pure commercial preparations contain all manner of nasty chemicals. If you use these receipts you'll know exactly what you're putting on your face and body and at the same time you'll be able to custom tailor each product to your own needs.

I really can't improve on the advice given in an 1870 beauty advice pamphlet: "... we feel safe in assuring the most careful & conservative mothers that the compounding at home and use of any of the preparations herein recommended will be a

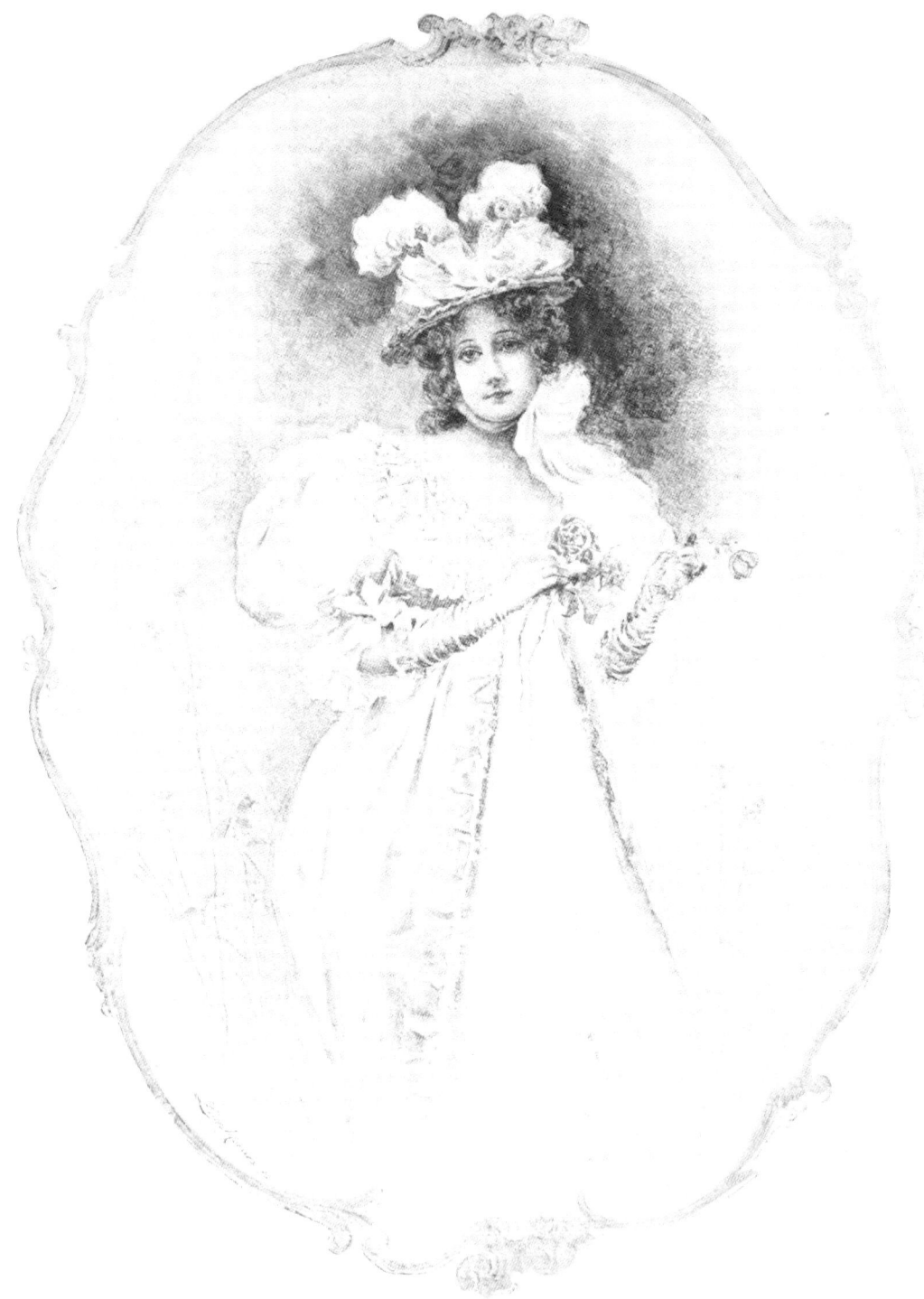

Oh Rose-leaf! flushing when the South
Doth woo thee with a warm caress,
Thy dainty hues enchant me less
Than Hebe's rosebud cheek and mouth;

For nothing ever can repair
Thy tender blushes when they fade;
But Hebe, happy little maid!
Hath Ivory Soap to keep her fair.

Copyright 1896, by The Procter & Gamble Co., Cin'ti.

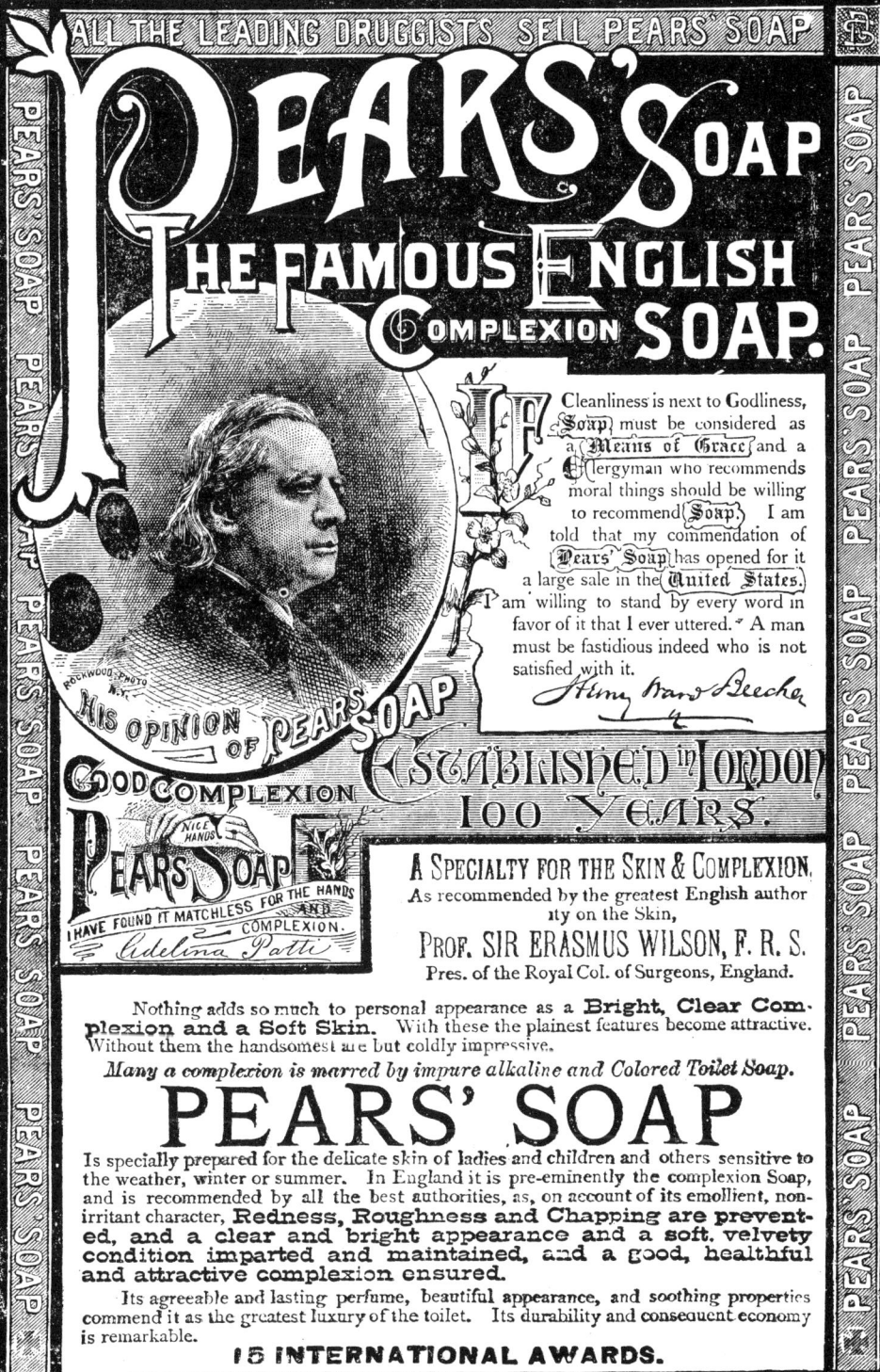

perfectly safe and innocent employment for their daughters or themselves. Any disposition to do so, we think, should be encouraged. A few vials of the essential oils, small quantities of almonds and other required ingredients, may be bought at the drugstore for less than a single bottle of the proprietary article can be purchased, and all interested will have the satisfaction of knowing that the materials are fresh and of good quality, and that no harmful consequences from their use need be feared."

All the receipts are based on old formulae, but in many cases I've altered them to take advantage of modern methods and equipment. The purpose of these preparations is to be able to make good, wholesome cosmetics, and if a blender does the job as well as "beating well in a wooden mortar for two or three hours" I've opted for the newfangled machinery rather than people-power!

Here are a few pointers which will make your efforts much easier and more predictable.

First, any of the pots or containers you use to make or store these cosmetics should be made of stainless steel, enamel, or glass. Aluminum or other metals are apt to react with the ingredients and spoil your results. Save old cosmetic containers and little jars to put your homemade goodies in, there's nothing worse than mixing up a batch of cream and realizing you have nothing to put it in. I find babyfood jars are an ideal solution.

When a receipt specifies the use of a double-boiler, I find a Pyrex measuring cup placed in a saucepan with about an inch of water in the pan is an ideal substitute, since most double-boilers are too big to conveniently hold the small amounts these receipts make.

When a receipt specifies a mixture should be filtered, I've found any of the coffee filters—Melitta, Chemex, or any of the paper filter brands—are perfect. Either use the paper filters in their holders or simply support the folded cone-shaped paper in the mouth of a jar.

Finally, any of these cosmetics will keep much better if they are refrigerated. Label them clearly so no one eats them by mistake!

Enjoy your natural cosmetics, and I'm sure you'll find that, like most of the receipts in this book, they make excellent gifts.

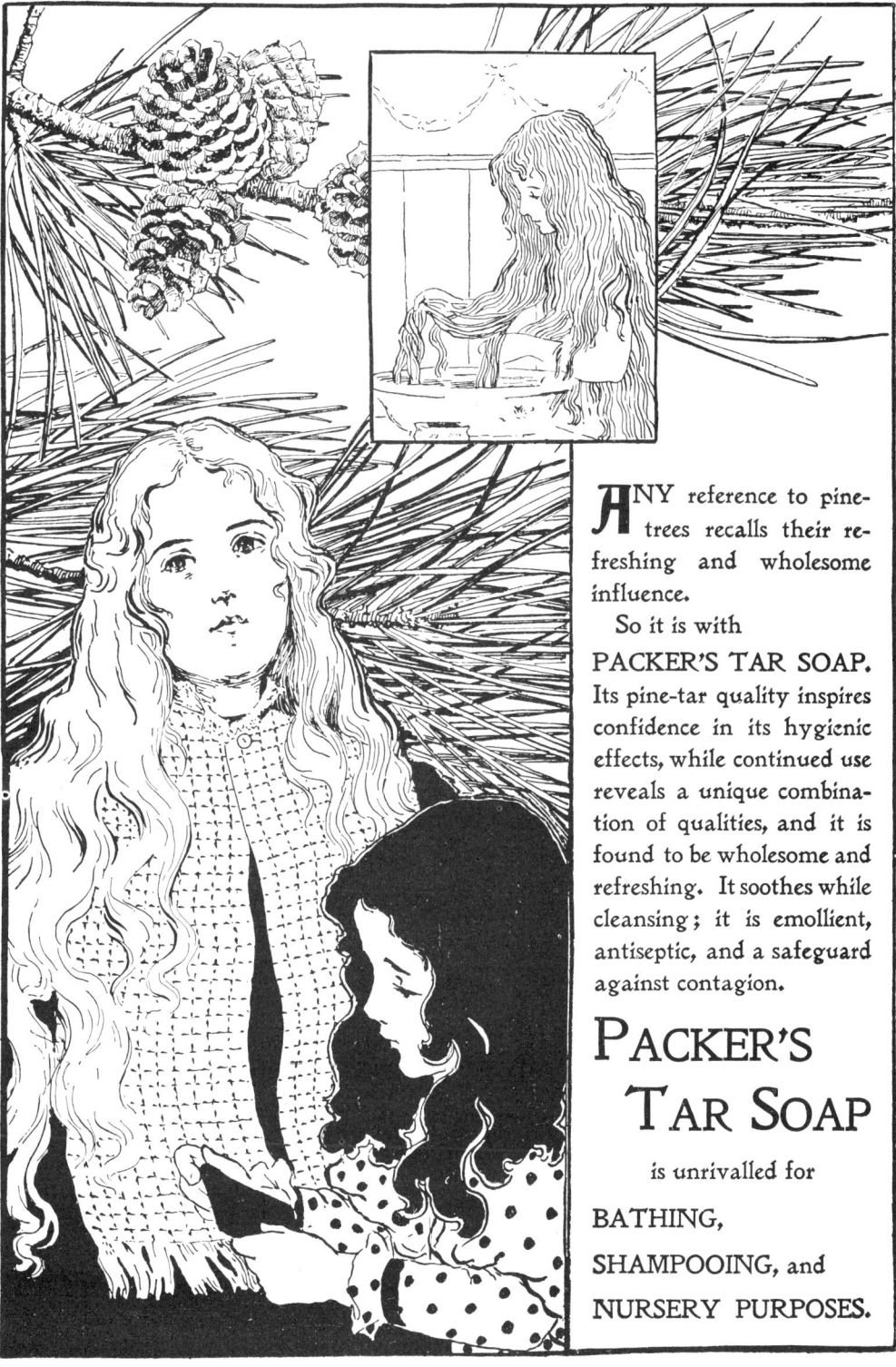

ANY reference to pine-trees recalls their refreshing and wholesome influence.

So it is with

PACKER'S TAR SOAP.

Its pine-tar quality inspires confidence in its hygienic effects, while continued use reveals a unique combination of qualities, and it is found to be wholesome and refreshing. It soothes while cleansing; it is emollient, antiseptic, and a safeguard against contagion.

PACKER'S TAR SOAP

is unrivalled for

BATHING,

SHAMPOOING, and

NURSERY PURPOSES.

Soaps, Creams & Facials

Making your own soap can be a very interesting hobby, and, with the rising price of "natural" soaps, money-saving too. The following receipt is an adaptation of colonial methods. Since we no longer have to make our own lye from wood ashes, and no longer have the need to make 200-pound batches, I've tailored the amounts and methods to the modern kitchen.

TO MAKE SOAP: Save all your cooking grease—bacon fat, drippings from fat roasts, and any other grease, oil or fat left over from cooking—until you have enough to render down to six pounds. (To render the fat simmer it with an equal amount of water until it is clear and all the solid matter has boiled to crisps. Then cool to room temperature until the fat solidifies, then skim it off with a slotted spoon, leaving the crisp bits and other mess with the water in the pot.) Take this rendered fat, and for every six pounds of fat you will need one pound of lye. Make sure the can specifies the lye is suitable for soapmaking—you *cannot use drain cleaners in its place!* Using an enamel pot dissolve each pound of lye in five cups of cold water. (Be very careful when working with lye. It can cause violent reactions and heat the water to boiling. I recommend wearing rubber gloves.) Warm the lye solution to 90°F, heat the fats to 110–125°F (use a candy thermometer to test the temperatures—they're crucial to your success). Slowly pour the lye solution in a steady dribble into the fats, stirring constantly, but not too vigorously. If you're too enthusiastic stirring, the soap will separate. Remove from the stove and continue gently stirring until the soap is the consistency of thick syrup. This will take about 15 minutes, and as soon as it's thickened you can add your own special ingredients.

The following are a few of my favorites:

    1 ounce powdered gum benzoin, 1/4 ounce oil of verbena, 10–15 drops of oil of vetiver. The result is a wonderful lemony soap which is slightly antiseptic due to the gum benzoin.

    1 ounce powdered gum benzoin, 1/4 to 1/2 cup honey, 1/4 ounce oil of jasmine, 5–10 drops of ambergris oil. A very sensuous-smelling soap.

    2 ounces orris powder, 1/8 ounce oil of lavender, 1 ounce powdered gum benzoin. A very clean-smelling soap. Store the

Good morning
Have you used PEARS' Soap?

bars in your linen closet while they're waiting to be used and your sheets and towels will take on a delightful aroma.

The other possibilities are: any of the scented oils, cornmeal, almond meal, oatmeal (for their abrasiveness), food coloring, powdered milk, ground vegetables or fruits, perfumes, etc. Just be careful not to add too much!

After you've added your extra ingredients, pour your soap into molds. I use a cardboard candy box lined with a damp cloth, but you can use any container that is flexible enough to get the soap out of after it's hardened. After twenty-four hours you can unmold your soap, and if you've used a box or other large container for the mold, cut it into bars. The soap now needs to be "cured," which simply means it needs to dry out and harden for at least two weeks. I let the bars harden a bit, then store them in my drawers and closets to make everything smell good.

(adaptation of colonial receipts)

The colonials were just as obsessed with wrinkles and impending old age as women are today. There are numerous receipts for wrinkle preventatives and removers, many of them seemingly more unpleasant than the wrinkles themselves! The following is one of my favorites, not as much for the receipt itself as for the author's comment.

TO REMOVE WRINKLES: Boil Gum Benzoin in Spirits of Wine till it forms a rich tincture. Put fifteen drops in a glass of water and use the resulting liquor to wash your face. Let it dry on the skin. It will obliterate wrinkles as far as anything can beside enamel.

(17th century receipt)

This particular wrinkle oil has been given rave reviews from everyone I've asked to try it. I imagine the honeysuckle bark contains some sort of natural astringent which tightens the skin, but whatever the active ingredient is, it sure seems to work.

HONEYSUCKLE WRINKLE OIL: Simmer on a very low fire or over water 1½ ounces of honeysuckle bark in 4 ounces of olive oil. Do this for one hour. Cool and strain through a fine cloth. Use on dry or wrinkled skin. You may scent this when cool with oil of honeysuckle or the scent of your choice.

(19th century receipt)

This is a wonderfully rich emollient cream which should really be a basic in your cupboard of natural cosmetics. If you have a favorite scent add a few drops along with the egg white. This has much better keeping qualities if refrigerated.

WRINKLE CHASER: Separate one egg, putting the yolk into a small jar with a tight-fitting cover and saving the white. Add 2 tablespoons of honey to the yolk and stir well until thick and smooth. Add the white, put on the cover, and shake *very* hard. When well-mixed you will have a thick, rich, smooth cream that is particularly well-suited for those wrinkled areas on the face and neck. If you add a few drops of tincture of benzoin it will last much longer without spoiling. In any case, this is best refrigerated.

(variation of a 19th century receipt)

The author of the following three wrinkle removers was undoubtedly a very taciturn New Englander who believed in getting right to the point with no embellishments!

TO REMOVE WRINKLES: Rub the face with Castor Oil before retiring

or

Rub the face with Almond Oil

or

Rub the face with fresh cream.

(*Peterson's National Ladies Magazine,* 1880)

Tinctures and oils of various flowers and vegetables were used to scent the colonials' cosmetics. Use your imagination—just about any scented botanical will do, and, by using the same process with such common items as lemon or orange peel, some truly unique fragrances are yours for very little effort or money. You don't have to mix them with these cosmetics to enjoy them; use them as is for a delightful cologne. (Also check the chapter on Herbs & Herb Compounds.)

TO PREPARE TINCTURES OF FLOWERS: A tincture of flowers having a strong perfume, as the tuberose, jasmine, violet, jonquil, and heliotrope, may be prepared by crowding fresh blossoms into a fruit jar and covering them with alcohol. After they have stood for a few days, the mixture may be strained through a linen cloth, the flowers squeezed to extract as much of the essence as possible, and fresh flowers added, and the process repeated until the desired strength is attained.

Or glycerin may be scented for the toilet and bath with any desired odor by the same method.

Or put half-inch layers of any flowers in an earthen pot or glass jar with layers of fine salt between. Screw the top on tightly and place the jar in a cellar or other dark, cool place. This process requires from one to two months. At the end of this time strain and squeeze the liquor through a cloth, put it into a glass bottle, and let it stand in the sun to clarify. Or place dry rose or other petals in a large bottle or fruit jar, cover with alcohol or other rectified spirits, close tightly, and preserve for use. A few drops of this tincture sprinkled about a room will give it a delicious perfume.

(*Household Discoveries*, 1882)

Here's another variation of the preceding receipt. I've included it because it's an ideal way to make use of those potted geraniums that have just about expired. Now you have a way to make that geranium live on!

GERANIUM PERFUME: A perfume which is very agreeable to many may be made by either of the above methods from the leaves of any of the sweet-smelling geraniums. The tincture, obtained by packing the leaves in a fruit jar, filling it with alcohol and allowing it to stand for a few weeks, is perhaps the easiest to prepare. The leaves may be renewed, if desired, to strengthen the perfume.

(*Household Discoveries*, 1882)

The colonials favored Bay Rum as an all-purpose scent, and even in the most masculine minds it was considered an acceptable toiletry. The following is my modified version, since the original receipts all utilize a still, which very few of us have in our kitchens today.

BAY RUM: Take a bottle with a tight-fitting cap that holds at least 6 ounces. Put into the jar the following ingredients: 4 ounces of 100 Proof Vodka, 1½ ounces of Dark Jamaican Rum, ¼ teaspoon of crushed allspice, 1 stick of cinnamon, 4 or 5 drops of oil of orange, a pinch of dried sage, a bit of lemon rind, a bit of lime rind, and a bit of orange rind (each about the size of a 50¢ piece). Put on the cap tightly and let it stand for 2 weeks, shaking daily. At the end of this period filter through filter paper and bottle for use.

(variation of an 18th century receipt)

This receipt is both a perfumed body oil and bath oil. You can substitute any oil you choose for the olive oil—my choice would be mink oil or oil of sweet almonds. And remember, cut down the quantities if four pounds of Oil of Roses is more than you can use (which I can almost guarantee it is)!

TO MAKE OYLE OF ROSES: Take a pound of red Rose buds, beat them in a marble morter with a wooden pestle, then put them in an earthen pot, and pour upon them four pound of Oyle of Olives, letting them infuse the space of a month in the Sunne, or in the chimney corner stirring of them sometimes, then heat it, and press it and strain it, and put it in the same pot or other vessel to keep.

(*The Charitable Physitian,* 1639)

This is the best solution ever for "dish-pan hands." Keep it by both the bathroom and kitchen sinks to use after every hand washing. (My choice of scent is usually a few drops of oil of lemon.) This is also a great favorite with those people who abstain from preparations containing animal products.

FRUIT OIL: In the top of a double-boiler melt together 1 ounce each of sweet almond oil, palm oil, persic oil, and olive oil; and ½ ounce of cocoa butter. When they are all nicely melted remove from the heat and add ¼ teaspoon tincture of benzoin, and then add a few drops of any scented oil of your choice. Pour into a bottle and cap well.

(variation of an 18th century receipt)

Here's a real classic cleanser/moisturizer that was a staple cosmetic from the time of the ancient Greeks. I've found a blender makes the job much easier and a tea strainer serves as an excellent sieve. This stuff is well worth the effort even if you do decide to use a mortar and pestle. Use this as a base for any number of additional ingredients— it's a perfect start for your own personalized line of cosmetics.

MILK OF ALMONDS: Rub up in a mortar 1 ounce of blanched almonds by adding, a little at a time, ½ pint of distilled water or pure soft water, mixing and rubbing constantly until a smooth, homogenous milky emulsion is formed. Finally strain the resulting mixture through a piece of net or gauze to remove the coarser particles. This is the common "Milk of Almonds" of perfumers, to which glycerin, various cosmetics, perfumes, and coloring matter may be added as desired.

(*Success Magazine,* 1868)

This receipt is for an especially good eye cream. Perfume it with a drop or two of your favorite scent to mask the odor of the lanolin—you'll have made a rich moisturizing cream that smells good, feels good, and is as good or better at its job than any commercial preparation.

RICH MOISTURIZING CREAM: Mix three ounces of pure lanolin with enough oil of sweet almonds to make a cream the consistency of cold cream. This is very good for the dry skin around the eyes, but it may be used wherever you need moisture—face, hands, elbows, et cetera.

(*Christian Herald & Signs of Our Times,* 1850)

Cucumber beauty treatments have been around for hundreds of years and recently they have gone through a great rebirth as the "in" organic skin aid. This receipt is an adaptation of a "Cucumber Beauty Milk" I found in an old journal. Cucumber juice is very perishable and this cosmetic *must* be refrigerated.

CUCUMBER MILK: Grate three or four large cucumbers (a blender is much easier, or better still, a vegetable juicer if you happen to have one), place them in a linen towel and squeeze as much juice out of them as you possibly can. Dilute with one half a cup of rosewater, a half-teaspoon of tincture of benzoin, and mix well. Use as a soothing facial rinse, especially good for raw and chapped skin.

(variation of an early 19th century receipt)

This concoction appears in 18th century almanacs right through 20th century household advice books. Any of the 100% bran cereals are suitable for use in this receipt.

BRAN FOR THE HANDS: Boil a small quantity of the bran in a cloth bag. Put both the juice and the boiled bran in the washbowl, add warm or hot water, and wash the hands with or without soap. This is perhaps the best and simplest treatment for the redness, dryness, and roughness caused by housework and exposure. After washing, the hands may be rubbed with a few drops of honey or a lotion composed of ¼ pound of honey, ½ pound of sal soda, and 1 pint water. Mix well and heat without boiling.

(*Household Advice,* 1840)

I think *everyone's* grandmother used this. It's perhaps the most basic and famous (not to mention enduring) of all the colonial toilet preparations. As effective as ever, it's really a delight to use.

 GLYCERIN & ROSEWATER: Mix together 3 ounces of glycerin with 7 ounces of rosewater. You may use any scented water in place of the rosewater (orange-flower, elder-flower, celery, camomile, etc.). Use to soften and comfort the hands.

(an 18th century receipt)

This is a richer, more complicated version of Glycerin & Rosewater. It's good to have on hand when you want a lotion that's more moisturizing and longer lasting than the preceding receipt. .

 AN EXCELLENT CREAM FOR THE HANDS: Take 3 ounces of lanolin, 1 ounce of sweet almond oil, 2 drams of glycerin, and 2 drams of rosewater. Use on the hands as often as possible and you are assured of beneficial results.

(an 18th century receipt)

For those of you who really feel like going all-out and are willing to take the time and effort, the following receipt makes a very elegant and professional product. It's much easier than baking a cake and you can enjoy the results every day for weeks. You may use just about any fruit or vegetable juice in place of the peach. Remember, you're not limited by anything but your own imagination! (This *must* be refrigerated!)

 PEACH LOTION: Thoroughly mash a peach and then strain the juice through a linen handkerchief or napkin, squeezing forcefully so as to extract all the juice. Add two ounces of coconut or almond oil, five drops tincture of benzoin, one and a half ounces of orange-flower water and one or two drops of oil of orange. Beat together until fluffy. Use to lubricate and moisturize your skin.

(a late 19th century receipt)

This receipt is very similar to Peach Lotion, but has more "substance" to it. As a matter of fact, it's so good I've often been tempted to eat it—and there's no reason why you couldn't as it contains no harmful ingredients! (Try that with one of your popular commercial brands—which means *don't*. To give you an idea of what you put on your body every day, here is a listing of the ingredients in one of those hair conditioners that you leave on after you shampoo: Water, Quaternium-18, Cetyl Alcohol, Glyceryl Stearate, Propylene Glycol Stearate SE, Isopropyl Alcohol, Formaldehyde, Fragrance, Color. Ugh! Nice of them to add fragrance and color as an afterthought.) So, come on, get out your strawberries and nice natural organic ingredients and get with it!

 STRAWBERRY CREAM: Mash and strain the juice from five or six

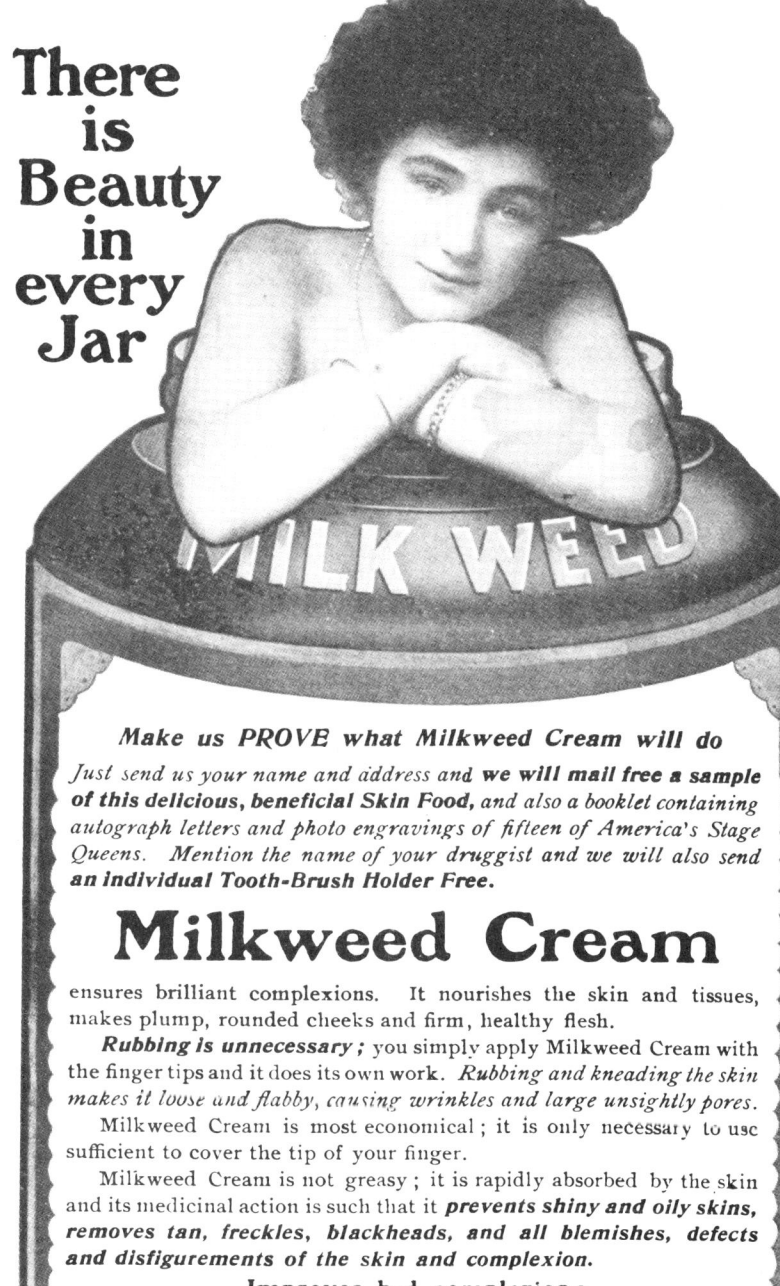

medium strawberries. Melt ½ an ounce of beeswax and 2½ ounces of coconut or sweet almond oil in a bain-marie. Remove from the heat and immediately add the strawberry juice. Beat the mixture until it is fluffy and *cool* or it will separate. Add three or four drops of tincture of benzoin and continue beating until thoroughly mixed.

(variation of a 19th century receipt)

Here's a cream that actually has cream in it. You'll find this is great to whip up in the summer for sunburn and that taught, dried-out feeling you get from too much sun. This will keep in the refrigerator for about a week.

PEACH CREAM: Mix 2 tablespoons of light cream with 2 tablespoons of fresh strained peach juice at room temperature. Add 6 tablespoons of very strong tea, again at room temperature, stirring constantly. When the tea is well-incorporated, slowly add 2 tablespoons of witch hazel, stirring constantly until the consistency is uniform and smooth.

(variation of a 19th century receipt)

Now on to the age-old adolescent problem—acne and pimples. This first receipt has been around as long as soap itself. (I got this version from my grandmother, who got it from *her* grandmother....)

TO DRY OUT PIMPLES AND/OR TO BRING THEM TO A HEAD: Brown or yellow laundry soap made into a paste with a little water and applied to the pimples and left on them will dry them out or bring them to a head.

(old family receipt)

This next receipt sounds as though it might *cause* pimples, but it really heals them up fast. I got this formula from a fancy New York dermatologist who found it in an 1830s doctor's manual.

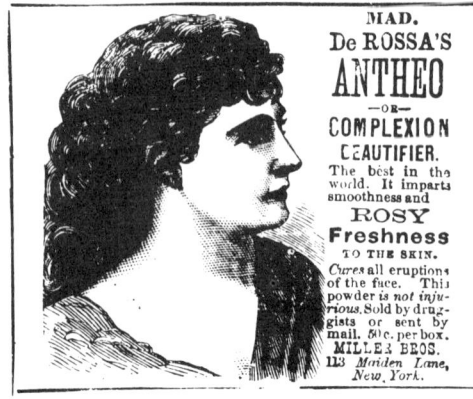

To Heal Pimples: Melt together equal quantities of lanolin, glycerin and castor oil. Mix well and pour into a jar with a well-fitting lid. Apply to pimples until healed.

(a doctor's manual, 1830s)

This treatment is a "facial scrub." All the abrasiveness, due to the almond meal and oatmeal, literally scrubs the pores clean and in the process gets rid of blackheads. Use this vigorously!

For Blackheads & to Refine the Pores: Mix together 16 ounces of uncooked powdered oatmeal, 8 ounces of almond meal, 4 ounces of powdered orris root, and 1 ounce of grated castile soap. Use as a facial wash.

(*Peterson's National Ladies Magazine,* 1868)

This is a much more passive treatment, but since tincture of benzoin is a very effective antiseptic there's good sense behind the mixture. I've found this is very good for those little inflammations that are more like a rash than actual pimples.

Kalydor: Dissolve 2 drams of tincture of benzoin in 1 pint of rosewater and use as a face wash for the complexion.

(*Household Discoveries,* 1882)

Now, on to those wonderful liquids known as astringents, herb waters, toilet vinegars, and facial stimulants. Their purpose is to rinse off all traces of cosmetics and dirt, and the following do that (and several other jobs) to perfection. This first rinse dates back to Elizabeth I and was a favorite of royalty right through Marie Antoinette. I found a more recent version in a 19th century ladies' magazine. This is a really great pick-me-up for an office-weary face, and the camphor's scent is a boost for your head.

To Tone the Skin: A few drops of Spirit of Camphor or a small piece of camphor ice in your facial rinse water will tone up the skin and put a glow to your complexion.

(*Peterson's National Ladies Magazine,* 1871)

This is a relatively strong astringent, due to the alum, but most people find it much milder than commerical products since it doesn't contain any alcohol. For added wallop store it in the refrigerator.

Herbal Astringent: Dissolve ¼ teaspoonful of alum in 3 tablespoonfuls of witch hazel, then add 4 tablespoonfuls of tincture of camomile, 1 teaspoonful of tincture of benzoin and a pinch of sage. Put into a well-closed bottle for 2 or 3 days, then filter and bottle.

(*Household Discoveries,* 1882)

These herbal vinegars are truly delightful. I imagine they evolved when some woman decided she wasn't going to make her tincture with alcohol and used vinegar instead. However they came about, they're soothing, wholesome, and exotic. And they really do help put your skin back to its normal Ph, which is destroyed by things like soap. So splash away and enjoy yourself!

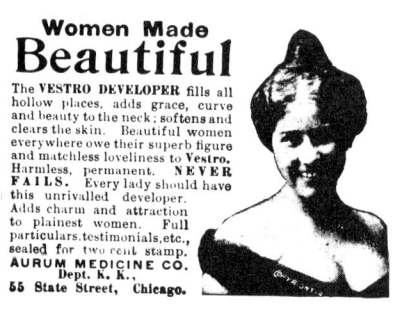

HYDRATING VINEGAR TO RESTORE THE SKIN'S NATURAL BALANCE: Combine ½ ounce of each of the following: orange flowers, orange peel, orange leaves, rose leaves, rose buds, rose hips, and camomile. Pour over them in a glass container 1 quart of good white wine vinegar, boiling. Cover the container and shake well daily until all the flowers and leaves have lost their color. Strain. Add 1 cup of orange or rosewater. Let settle for a week or two, then filter. A most excellent vinegar to use as an astringent, hair rinse, or body wash.

(variation of an 18th century receipt)

Here's a less complicated vinegar, but don't think that means it's "less good" than the preceding receipt. I happen to prefer this version, not only because it's easier to make but because I prefer the scent of just roses.

ROSE VINEGAR: Steep one ounce each of rose petals and chamomile flowers in two cups of white wine vinegar for at least two weeks. Strain and add one cup of rosewater. Dip a piece of absorbent cotton in the rose vinegar and use as an astringent wash for the face or body.

(variation of an 18th century receipt)

Here's an astringent that contains 50% alcohol—a combination that is much closer to today's astringents.

ROSEWATER ASTRINGENT: Mix equal quantities of rosewater and 50% grain alcohol. Use as a facial rinse on a piece of absorbent cotton.

(variation of a 19th century receipt)

This Apple Refresher is a good old-fashioned creation that's very good to use before applying your makeup base. I've also found it is very good for problem teenage skin... it makes skin happy!

APPLE REFRESHER: Mix together in a jar with a close-fitting top 2/3 cup of apple juice or sweet cider, 1/3 cup of 150 Proof Rum or Vodka, and 1/3 cup of witch hazel. Shake together. Use as a facial rinse, applied with the hands or a piece of absorbent cotton.

(variation of a 19th century receipt)

And now on to facial masks—those gooey preparations you smear on your face and leave there for a certain amount of time. They're the oldest cosmetic treatments we know of and they definitely predate any of the cosmetics we know today. Facials are excellent for refining pores, getting rid of blackheads, and tightening the skin. Colonial women had many ingredients at their disposal and by all accounts took advantage of them. Perhaps the simplest and most available was the egg facial: Simply take the white of an egg and smear it on your face and forehead. Wait fifteen minutes to a half hour, wash off, and your skin is smooth and taut and healthy looking. But let's go on to some slightly more complicated concoctions like

    EGG WHITE & HONEY FACIAL: Beat an egg white very stiff and add one tablespoonful of honey. Beat the honey in well until the mixture has the consistency of very thick whipped cream. Spread on the face and leave for at least 15 minutes. Rinse off well with cool water. Use once a week for best results.

                                                (variation of an 18th century receipt)

This mask is very good for oily skin and blackheads. It also makes any type skin very smooth and soft.

    A MASK: Take equal amounts of uncooked oatmeal and cornmeal and mix with rosewater or regular water to a thick spreadable texture. Place on the face and leave for at least half an hour. Wash off and rinse well.

An early ladies' magazine had this to say about cosmetic treatments: "The humblest meals afford the average woman reliable and inexpensive methods for preserving her good looks if she possesses the wish to make use of these lowly agents. Cornmeal and oatmeal retain heat for a great length of time. When mixed with very hot water and applied to the face and neck as poultices, they draw out impurities, and make very valuable bleaching masks, especially if lemon juice is added...

This mask is good enough to eat!

    HONEY & AVOCADO PEAR FACIAL: Whip together 1 tablespoon of mashed avocado pear, 2 tablespoons raw honey, and 2 egg whites or 1 whole egg until smooth. Spread freely on the face and leave there for 10 minutes. Rinse off thoroughly and your skin will be taut and smooth.

                                                (variation of a 19th century receipt)

You can use any of the many dairy products available in this receipt, but yoghurt, buttermilk, and heavy cream give the best results.

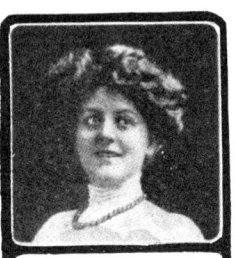

"Just a gleam of ivory in her smile"

Miss Adele Ritchie

one of America's most beautiful artistes, says:

"Zodenta will impart a radiance of dazzling white to the teeth that no other dentifrice can give."

ZODENTA
FOR THE TEETH

is different from all other dentifrices. Zodenta has the peculiar and special property of *dissolving all injurious deposits.* These deposits discolor and destroy the delicate enamel and cause what we know as "decayed teeth." It also *prevents the formation of tartar,* and its antiseptic and germicidal properties destroy *all poisons and germs* which cause *softened and diseased gums.*

Price 25c at all druggists

FREE

to every user of Zodenta a 7-inch oxidized silver Hat Pin. Send us the screw cap from the tube of Zodenta you buy at your drug store. If your druggist is out of Zodenta mail us 25c and mention the Hat Pin offer and we will send you the Zodenta and the Hat Pin, post-paid.

**F. F. INGRAM & CO.,
48 Tenth Street,
Detroit, Mich.**

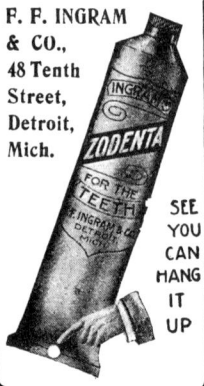

SEE YOU CAN HANG IT UP

A TREATMENT FOR THE FACE: Use yoghurt with a few drops of fresh lemon juice. Let it stay on for ten-twenty minutes. Rinse off and follow with rose or orange-flower water.

(*Household Discoveries,* 1882)

Why not experiment with your own personal facial, specifically formulated for your skin's needs. If one of the preceding receipts isn't quite right, try almond meal moistened with cucumber juice, buttermilk or rosewater. Or try almond meal moistened with plain water if your skin is very oily. The possibilities are endless and the end result will be a much better-looking you.

Ever since I found out the majority of toothpastes and mouthwashes contain formaldehyde I've been searching for a natural, effective substitute. The good colonial stand-bys—charcoal powder and salt or bicarbonate of soda—work well, but I went on in search of something more flavorful and exotic. I've had to modify the colonial receipts since they contain some ingredients that have been found to be harmful, or some which are no longer available. (One receipt called for oyster shells pounded to a fine powder in a mortar. I tried to reduce some oyster shells to a fine powder in a mortar and many hours later I ended up with a bagful of oyster shells reduced to a powder the texture of very coarse gravel. Either oyster shells have gotten harder or the colonials had some sort of knack for pounding things to a powder.) So my modifications to these old receipts have been made with the intention of improving on the originals while still maintaining their historical and esthetic accuracy. Try them. They're a very pleasant change from those chemical tasting pastes, and they have a very substantial bonus—you can drink an acid beverage like orange juice immediately after cleaning your teeth and experience none of that horrible aftertaste left by commercial preparations.

A TOOTH POWDER: Take one ounce of powdered myrrh, a pinch of powdered sage or mint, and two teaspoons of honey. Use to brush your teeth.

(variation of an 18th century receipt)

A TOOTH WASH: Brush your teeth with powdered charcoal moistened with honey. This will leave your teeth white and your mouth clean and fresh.

(a 17th century receipt)

MINT FLAVOURED MOUTH CLEANSER: Soak ¼ ounce of each of the following in ¾ cup of the strongest rum you can get: spearmint leaves, thyme leaves, crushed myrrh, and crushed cloves. Shake daily for a week and strain. Add ten drops of oil of peppermint. To be used diluted—one part of the above mixture to five parts of water. Rinse your mouth and gargle.

(variation of a 19th century receipt)

A great many of the colonials' hair preparations simply aren't suitable for today, but among the ones that are there are some very good ones indeed. The current craze for protein-enriched shampoos, setting lotions and rinses isn't all that revolutionary—the colonials made an infusion of beef marrow and used it as a hair treatment to be left on for about an hour and then rinsed out. Though I haven't been able to find a suitable period receipt for this treatment, the following is an approximation of the ones they used and is very good for giving body to fine hair.

MARROW HAIR TREATMENT: Take the marrow from one large marrow bone which your butcher has previously cracked and split. Mix with one ounce of olive oil and a few drops of rose oil. Put into your blender and blend at low speed for one minute. Apply to your hair, making sure to distribute it evenly over the entire scalp and to all your hair. Wrap your head with a towel which has been wet with as hot water as you can stand and then wrung out. Leave on your hair for 30-45 minutes, then wash your hair with a mild shampoo.

Here's another protein treatment that's much easier.

BEER SHAMPOO: Take one cup of beer and boil it until it has reduced to ¼ cup. Cool and add to your favorite shampoo.

(*Peterson's National Ladies Magazine*, 1870)

You can also take advantage of the benefits of beer by using stale beer right from the bottle as a setting lotion. It doesn't leave any odor and leaves the hair with added body and highlights. The colonials used bear grease as a treatment for dry, lifeless hair. If you'd like to try it, the following method is the most effective: At night rub a small amount of the bear grease through your hair and scalp. Put on a nightcap or wrap your head with a light towel and pin securely. In the morning, shampoo. Do as often as necessary, generally once every two weeks is sufficient. You can substitute a number of other preparations in place of the bear grease—castor oil, olive oil, mink oil and coconut oil are a few of the possibilities.

The colonials had all sorts of ingenious beauty tricks, many firmly rooted in the traditions they brought from the Old World, others indigenous to their new country. This treatment, in conjunction with a leisurely facial, will make you look healthy and rested in all but the most dire circumstances.

For Tired, Puffy Eyes: Brew some tea in a bit of rosewater. Cool. Moisten two cotton pads in the resulting liquor and place over the eyes. Leave on for fifteen minutes and the eyes will be clear and the skin around them firm. This treatment is even further improved with camomile flowers used in place of the tea.

(*Household Advice,* 1869)

With the current publicity about the dangers of talc containing asbestos particles, why not take advantage of an old substitute and use arrowroot powder instead. You can also use corn starch or powdered orris root. Here's a receipt for "A Sweet Powder" which is talc-free, beautifully scented, and fun to make.

A Sweet Powder: Take 5 ounces of powdered orris root, 2 ounces of powdered calamus, 2 ounces of powdered gum of benzoin, ½ ounce of powdered lavender buds, ¼ ounce of powdered cloves and 1 ounce of powdered rose petals. Mix all the ingredients together thoroughly and strain through a fine sieve, discarding any of the large particles that remain in the sieve.

(variation of an 18th century receipt)

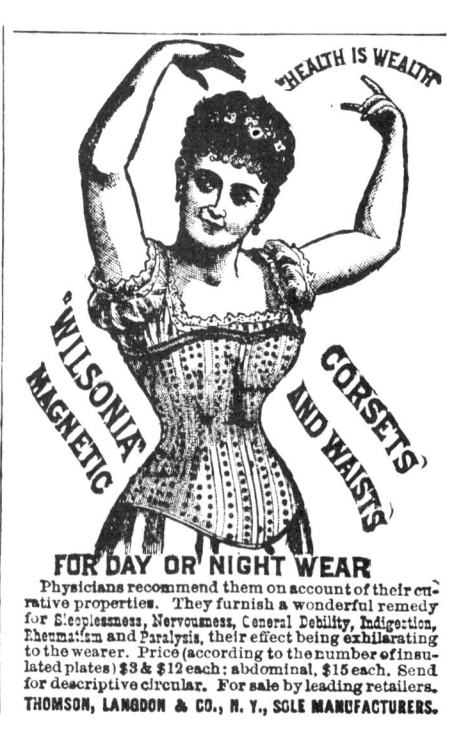

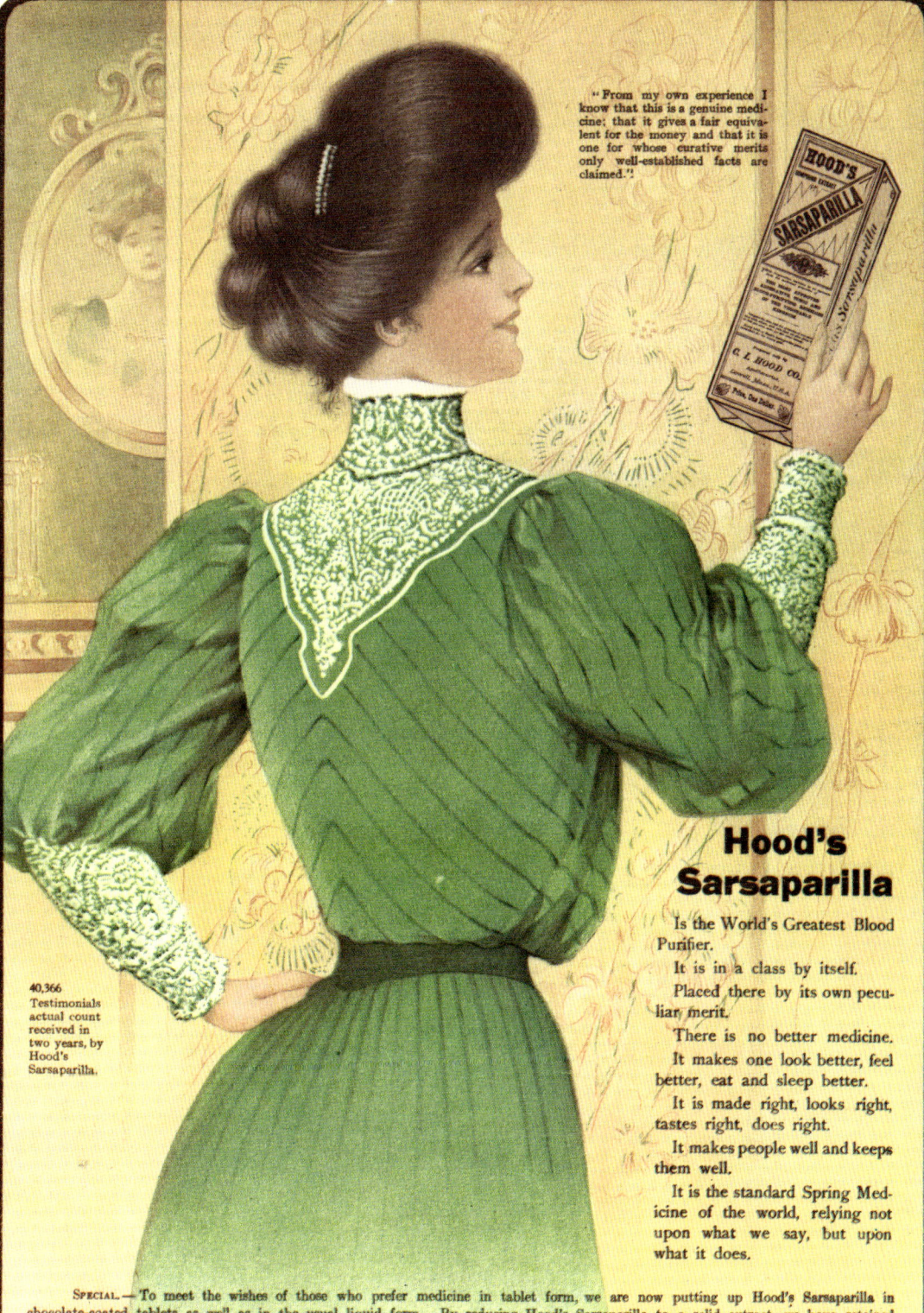

"From my own experience I know that this is a genuine medicine; that it gives a fair equivalent for the money and that it is one for whose curative merits only well-established facts are claimed."

40,366 Testimonials actual count received in two years, by Hood's Sarsaparilla.

Hood's Sarsaparilla

Is the World's Greatest Blood Purifier.

It is in a class by itself.

Placed there by its own peculiar merit.

There is no better medicine.

It makes one look better, feel better, eat and sleep better.

It is made right, looks right, tastes right, does right.

It makes people well and keeps them well.

It is the standard Spring Medicine of the world, relying not upon what we say, but upon what it does.

SPECIAL.— To meet the wishes of those who prefer medicine in tablet form, we are now putting up Hood's Sarsaparilla in chocolate-coated tablets as well as in the usual liquid form. By reducing Hood's Sarsaparilla to a solid extract, we have retained in the tablets the curative properties of every medicinal ingredient. Sold by druggists or sent by mail. 100 doses one dollar. C. I. Hood Co., Lowell, Mass. There is no substitute for Hood's Sarsaparilla because it is "Peculiar to Itself."

A SUMMER TONIC
Horsford's
ACID PHOSPHATE

A SIMPLE PRESCRIPTION

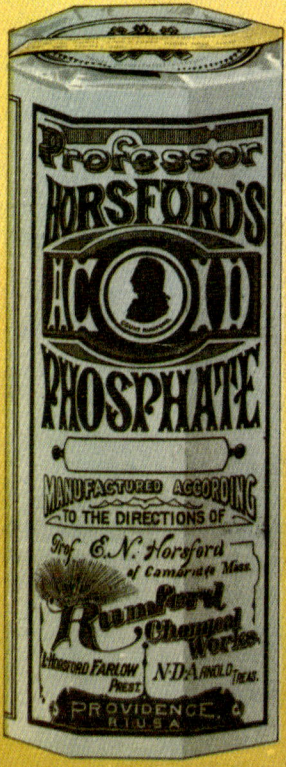

℞ When exhausted depressed or weary from <u>overwork</u> of mind or body take half a teaspoonful of *Horsford's Acid Phosphate* in half a glass of water

IF YOUR DRUGGIST CANNOT SUPPLY YOU, WE WILL SEND, POSTAGE PAID A TRIAL SIZE BOTTLE ON RECEIPT OF 25 CENTS

RUMFORD CHEMICAL WORKS, Providence, R.I.

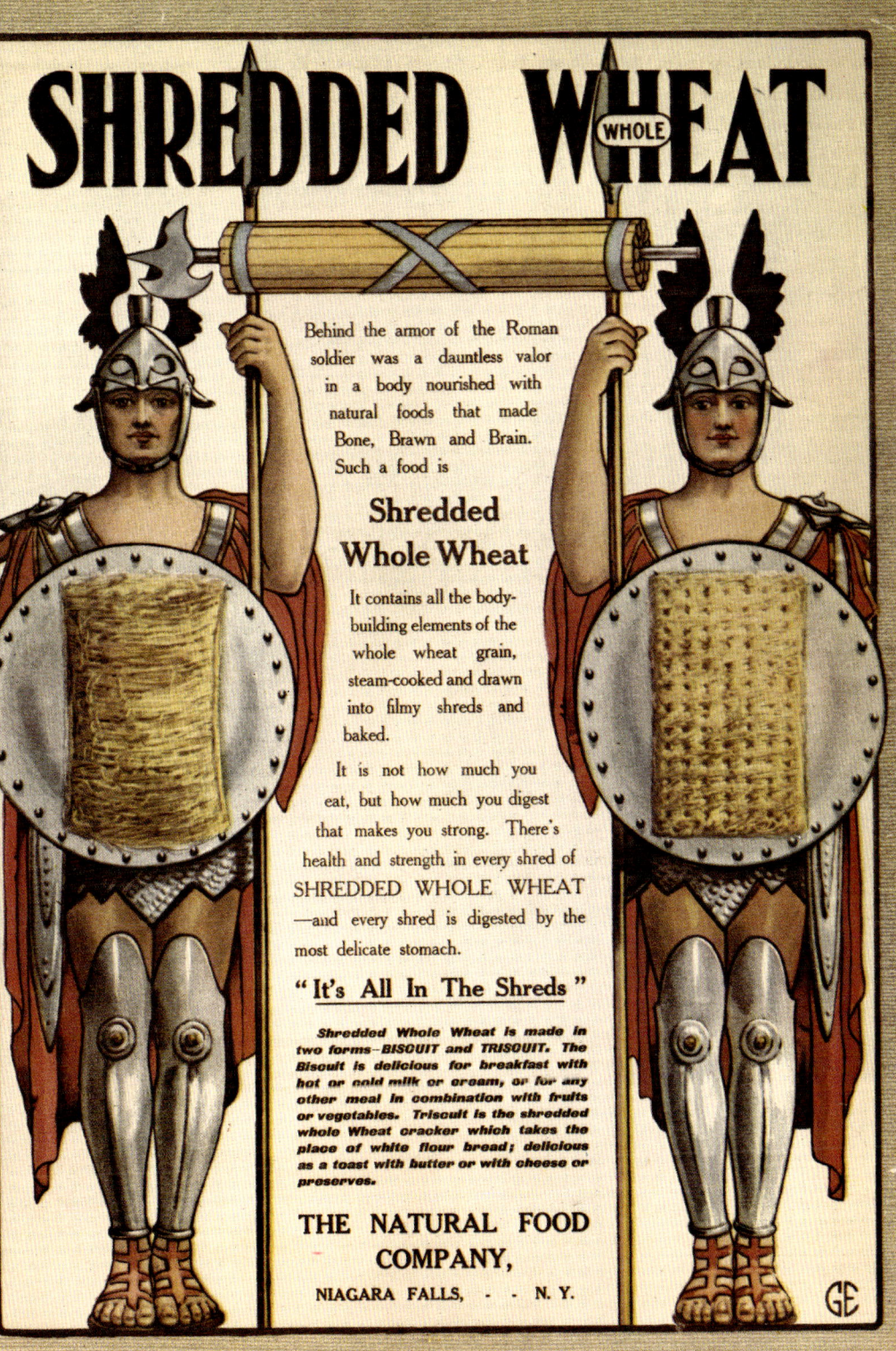

The Harmless Remedy For Headache and All Pain

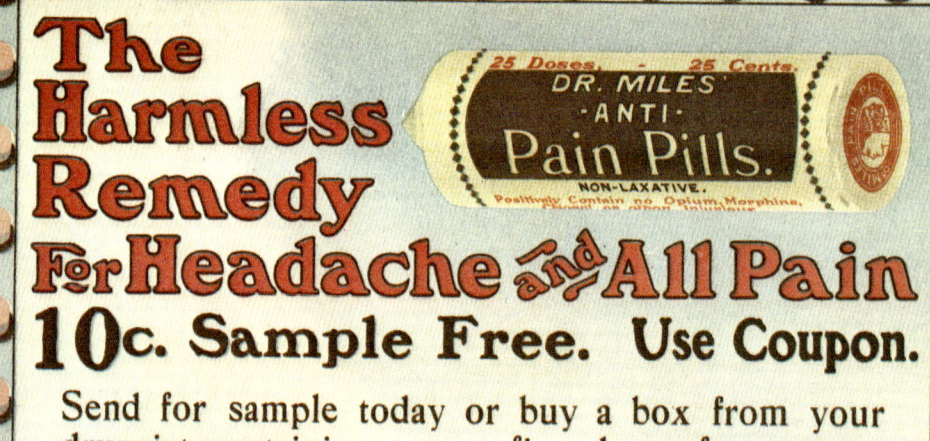

10c. Sample Free. Use Coupon.

Send for sample today or buy a box from your druggist containing twenty-five doses for twenty-five cents. They are put up in twenty-five cent size boxes only and are NEVER SOLD IN BULK.

Dr. Miles' Anti-Pain Pills are used and sold in every City, Town and Hamlet in the United States, and are considered the very best remedy for the relief of pain by all who use them. In addition to their wonderful curative properties, they have the added merit of being absolutely harmless when taken as directed.

Dr. Miles' Anti-Pain Pills do not contain opium, morphine, chloral, cocaine or similar dangerous drugs, and have no evil effect upon the system, nor tend to depress the Heart, if used as directed.

They are easy to take, and may be swallowed whole, chewed and swallowed, or taken dissolved in water with equally good results.

They are quick in action, **relieving headache in a few minutes,** while nearly every other form of pain readily yields to their magic influence.

They are safe, never causing nausea, vomiting or derangement of the stomach.

They do not affect the bowels in the slightest degree. Delicate women who suffer from sleeplessness, backache, bearing-down and other pains, find in them a pleasant and sure relief.

Their form is such that a few can always be carried in the pocket ready for immediate use upon the first approach of headache. Thousands of persons are thus enabled to travel, attend church or places of amusement, without the fear of headache, dizziness, car-sickness, nervousness, etc. They are a superior remedy for

Headache,	Irritability,	Backache,	Bearing-Down
Sciatica,	Sleeplessness,	Neuralgia,	Pains,
Rheumatism,	Blues,	Stomachache,	Etc., Etc.
Nervousness,	Seasickness,	Dizziness,	

The following literature is free by postal request: (1) Dr. Miles' 1905 U. S. Weather Almanac and Handbook of Valuable Information; (2) Know Your Heart; (3) Character of Faces; (4) The Nervous System; (5) What's Wrong; (6) What to Eat; (7) Story of Hands; (8) Only a Pain Pill; (9) Beautiful Illustrated 1905 Wall Calendar. Order by number, only one selection free, all of the books by sending two stamps to Dr. Miles Medical Company, Elkhart, Ind.

MILES MEDICAL CO., Elkhart, Ind.
Gentlemen: Please send me your free ten-cent sample package of Dr. Miles' Anti-Pain Pills.

Name:
Address:

Dr. MILES'
ANTI-PAIN PILLS
CURE HEADACHE AND RELIEVE ALL PAIN

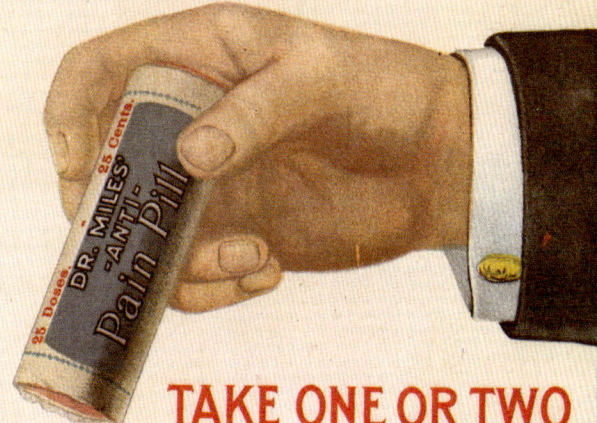

FOR SALE BY DRUGGISTS EVERYWHERE 25 DOSES, 25 CENTS. NEVER SOLD IN BULK

TAKE ONE OR TWO AND THE PAIN IS GONE

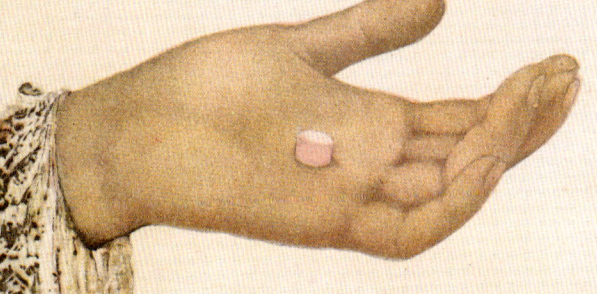

Postal Brings Sample Package, Free
MILES MEDICAL CO., ELKHART, IND.

DR. MILES' NERVINE

Makes Weak Nerves Strong

Allays Irritation and Nervousness
Brings Restful, Refreshing Sleep
Restores Strength and Vigor to the Tired, Worn-Out System

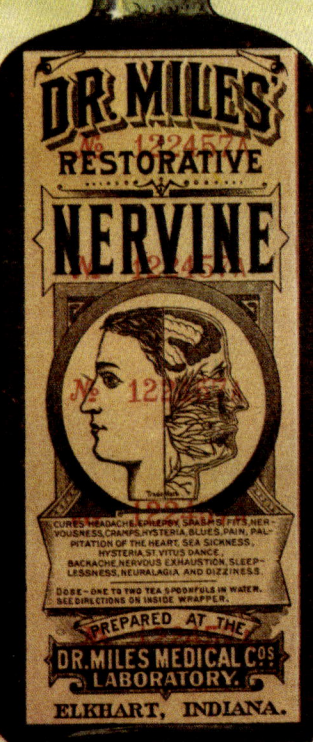

Dr. Miles' Restorative Nervine has been sold strictly on its merits for 30 years.

We believe it to be the best Remedy for all forms of Nervous Diseases.

We are so certain that it will help you that we authorize druggists to return the price of the first bottle if it fails to benefit.

One bottle will prove whether it will benefit your case; if not, you get your money back.

Try it on this proposition for Nervousness, Sleeplessness, Headache, Backache, Neuralgia, Nervous Prostration, Spasms, Fits, Epilepsy, Hysteria, Blues, Melancholy, Palpitation of the Heart and Stomach Troubles.

Sold by druggists everywhere--$1.00 per bottle.

FREE SAMPLE—A small bottle will be sent free on request. Address postal card to

Miles Medical Company,
Elkhart, Indiana.

Dr. Miles' Restorative Nervine contains no opium, chloral, cocaine, morphine or other harmful drugs.

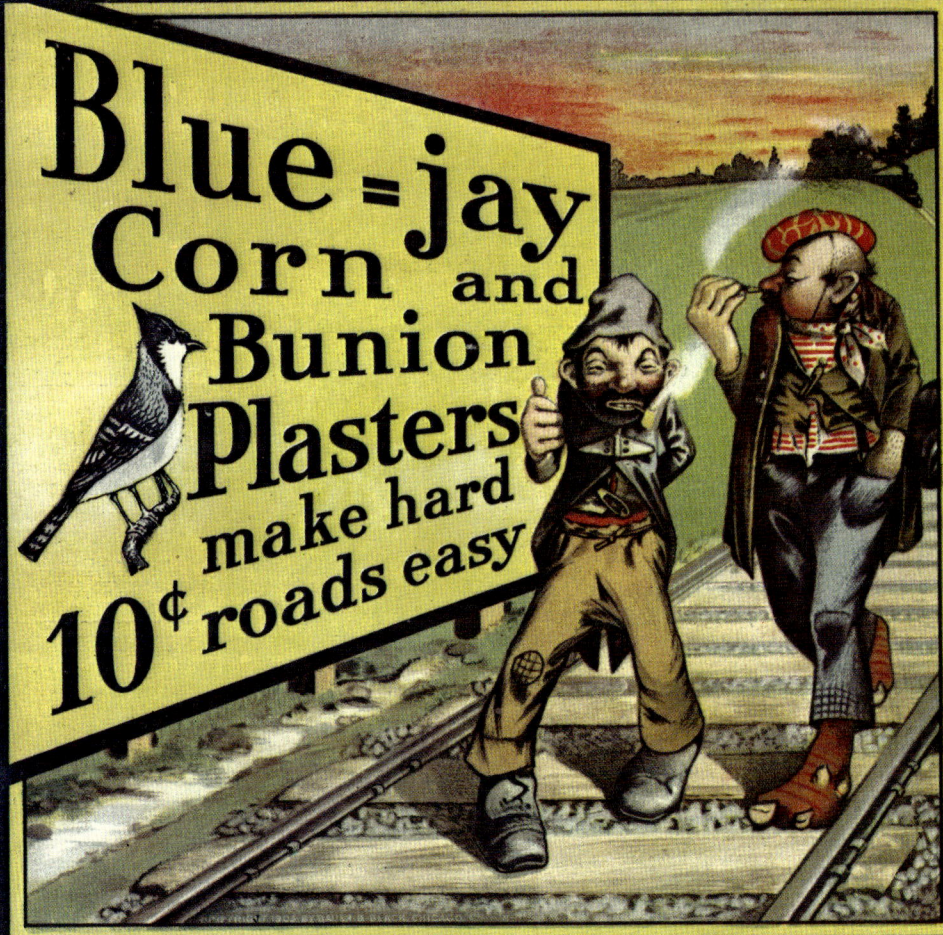

They Stop the Pain Instantly and Remove the Corn in 48 Hours

BLUE-JAY Corn and Bunion Plasters are made with a medicated center and a protecting ring of soft felt. An adhesive band holds the medication and the protecting ring firmly in place. They are easily and quickly applied—conform perfectly to the outlines of the toe or foot and give immediate ease and comfort. No uncleanly salves, liquids or clumsy bandages to bother with.

The secret of Blue-jay is that it takes out the corn—root and all—without pain or discomfort. No other corn plaster does this

If you cannot procure Blue-jay at the drug store, send us 10c. for a package of four corn plasters (enough for four corns). Bunion plasters, two in a package.

"Make Hard Roads Easy" is the title of a booklet which tells how to care for and treat the feet. It explains how to do chiropody at home and is invaluable to everyone troubled in any way with the feet. The booklet is free.

Bauer & Black, 287 25th Street, Chicago, U. S. A.

Makers also of Rex Porous Plasters, Mother's Mustard Plasters, Everybody's Court Plaster, Reed's Rubber Adhesive Plaster, Jap Tooth Silk, Handy Package Absorbent Cotton, Ford's Menthol Inhaler, Frost King and Frost Queen Chamois Vests.

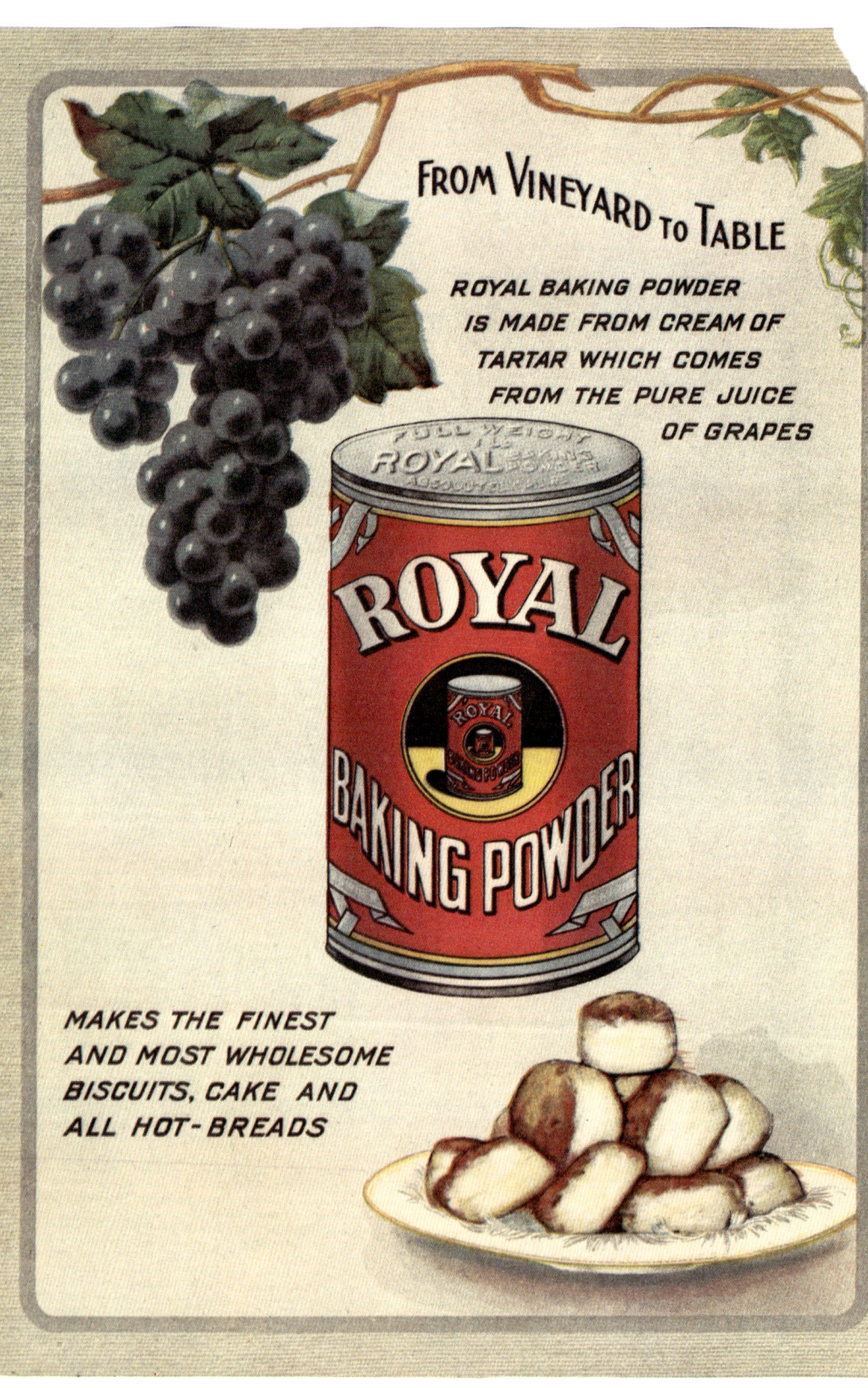

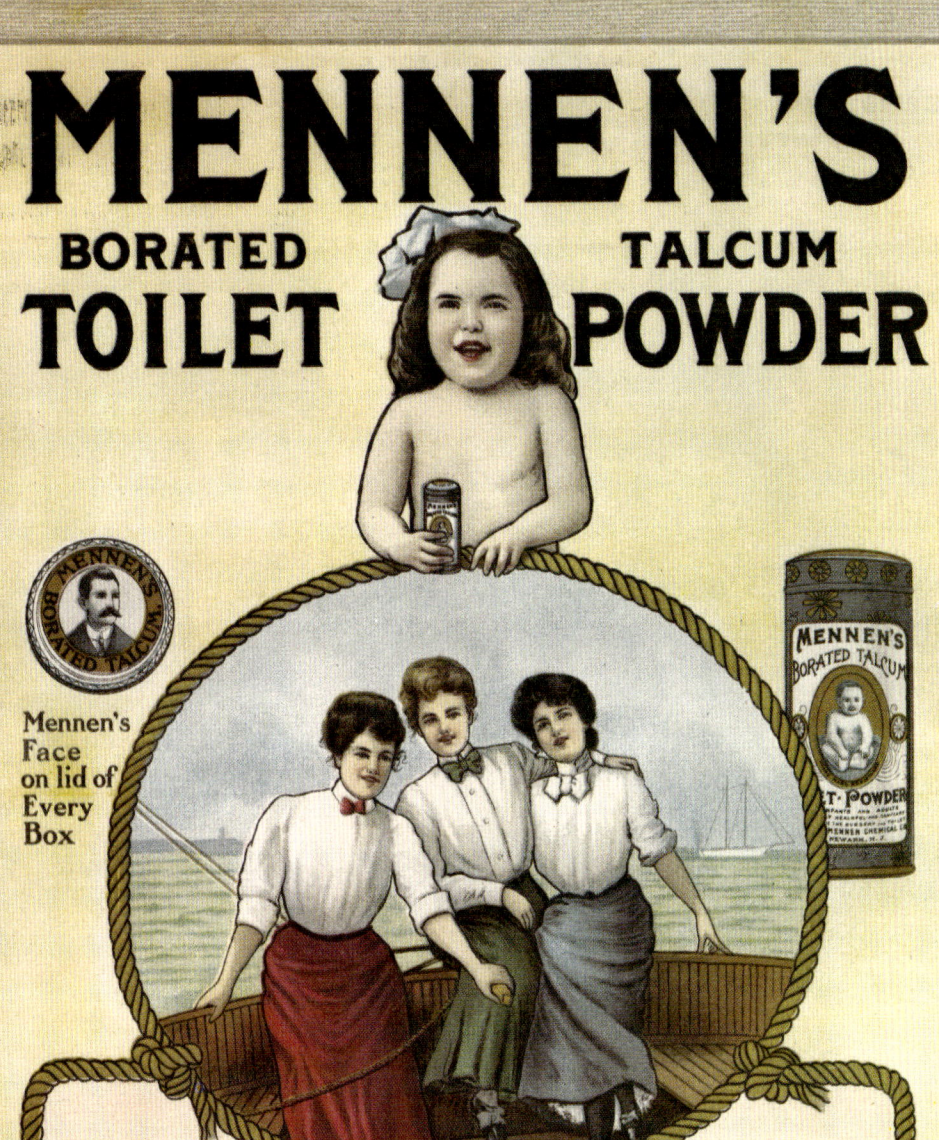

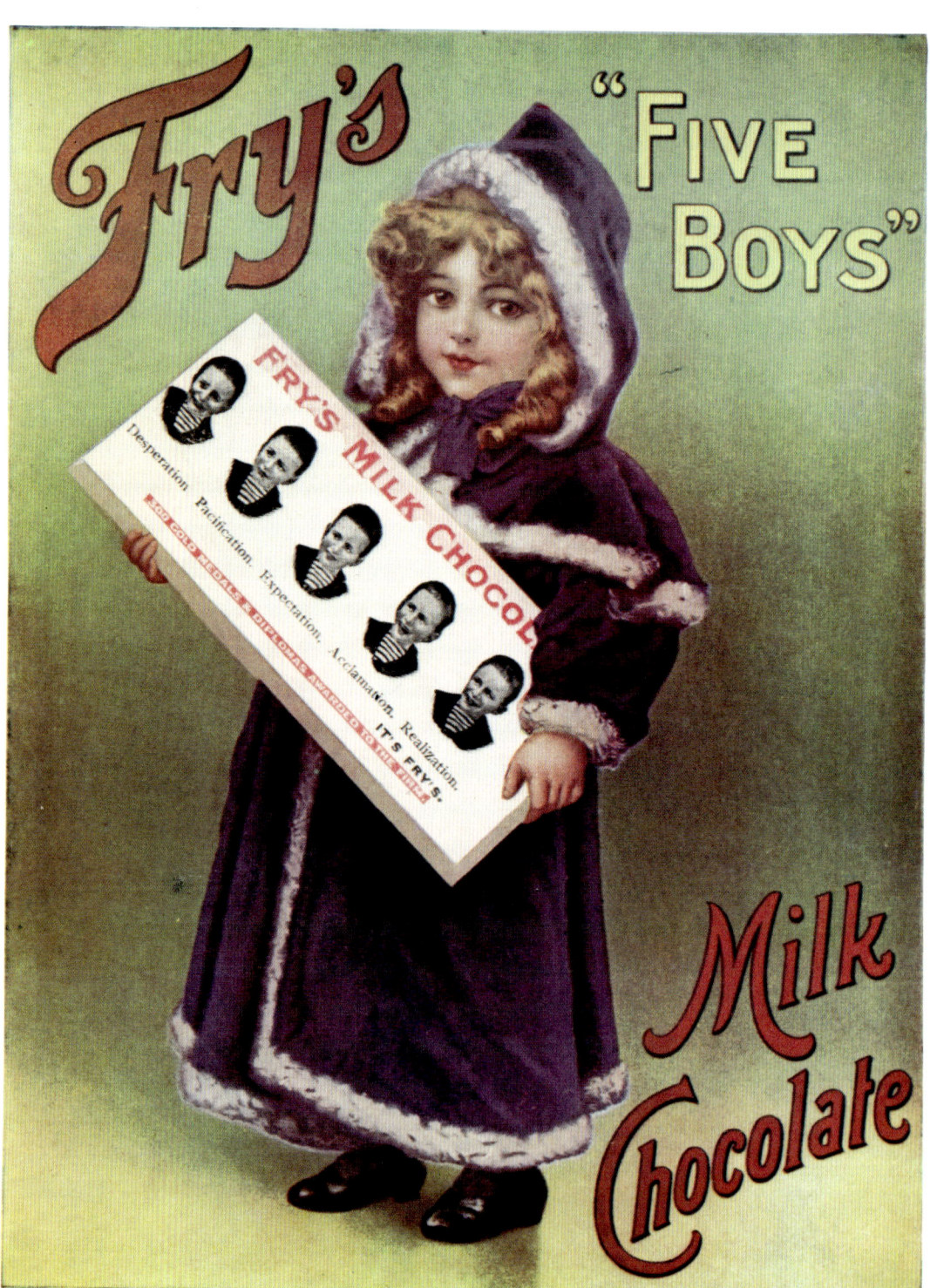

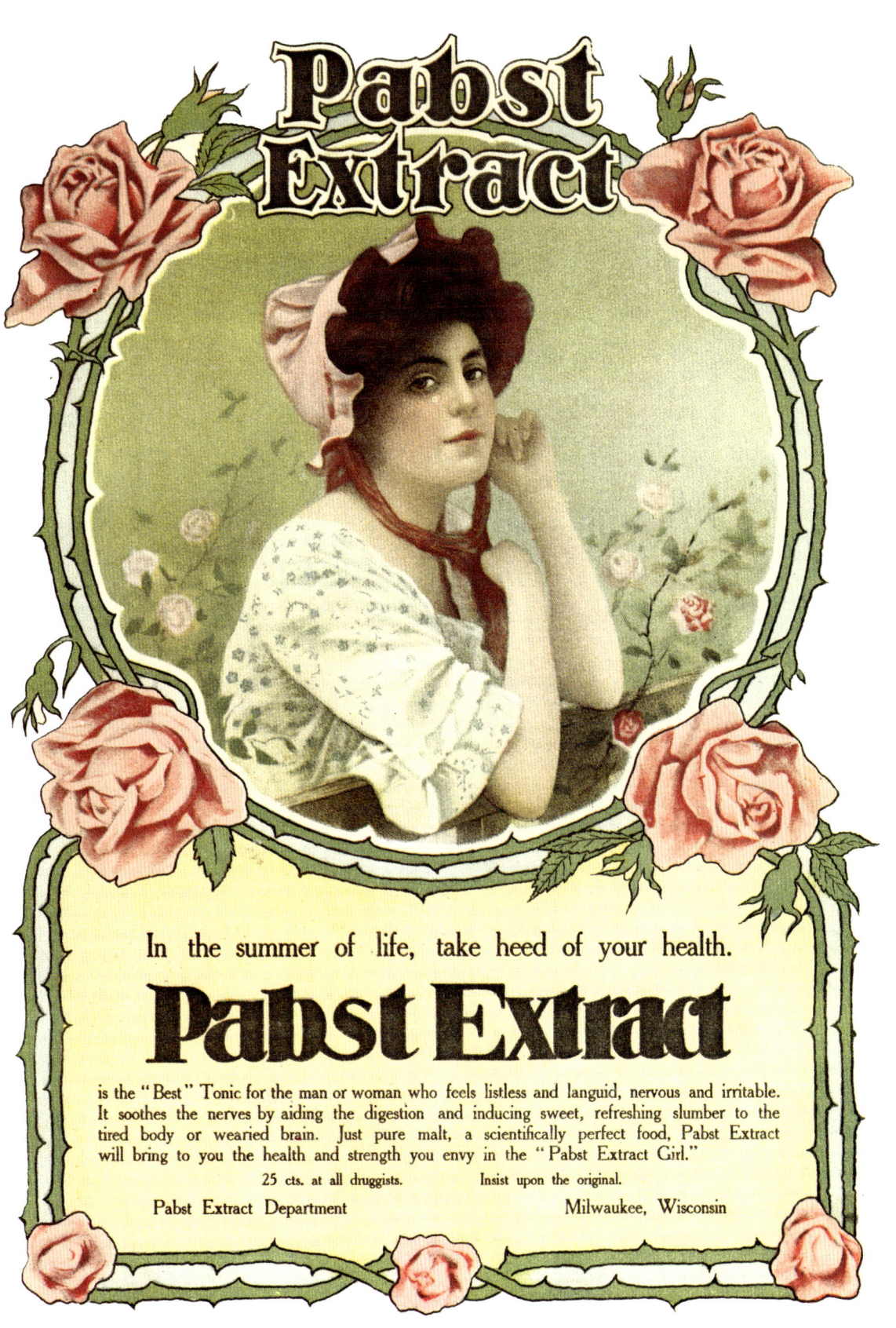

COMPLIMENTS OF
P. J. DEVITT,
Dealer in Boots & Shoes,
412 Main St., Bridgeport, Conn.
4

Compliments of
The Great A&P
Tea Co

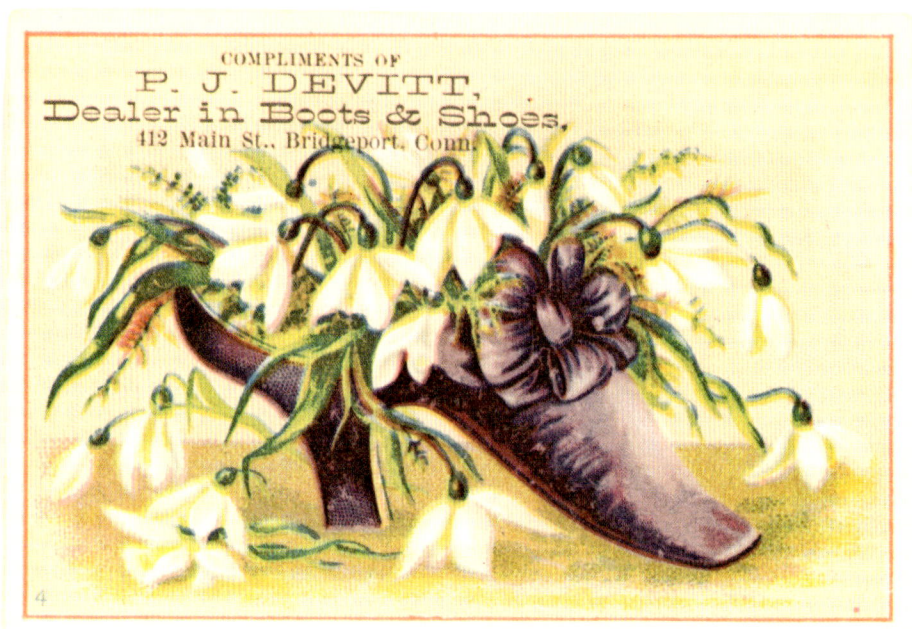

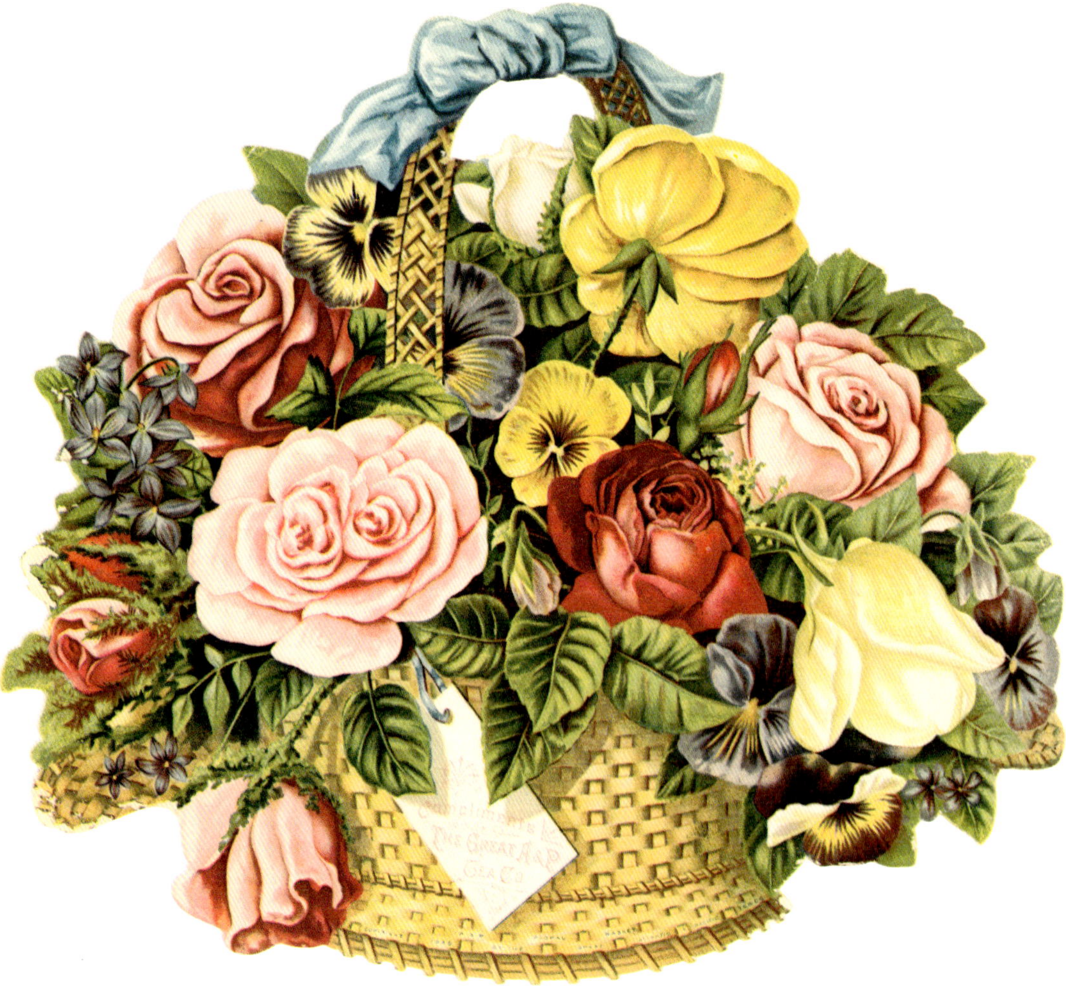

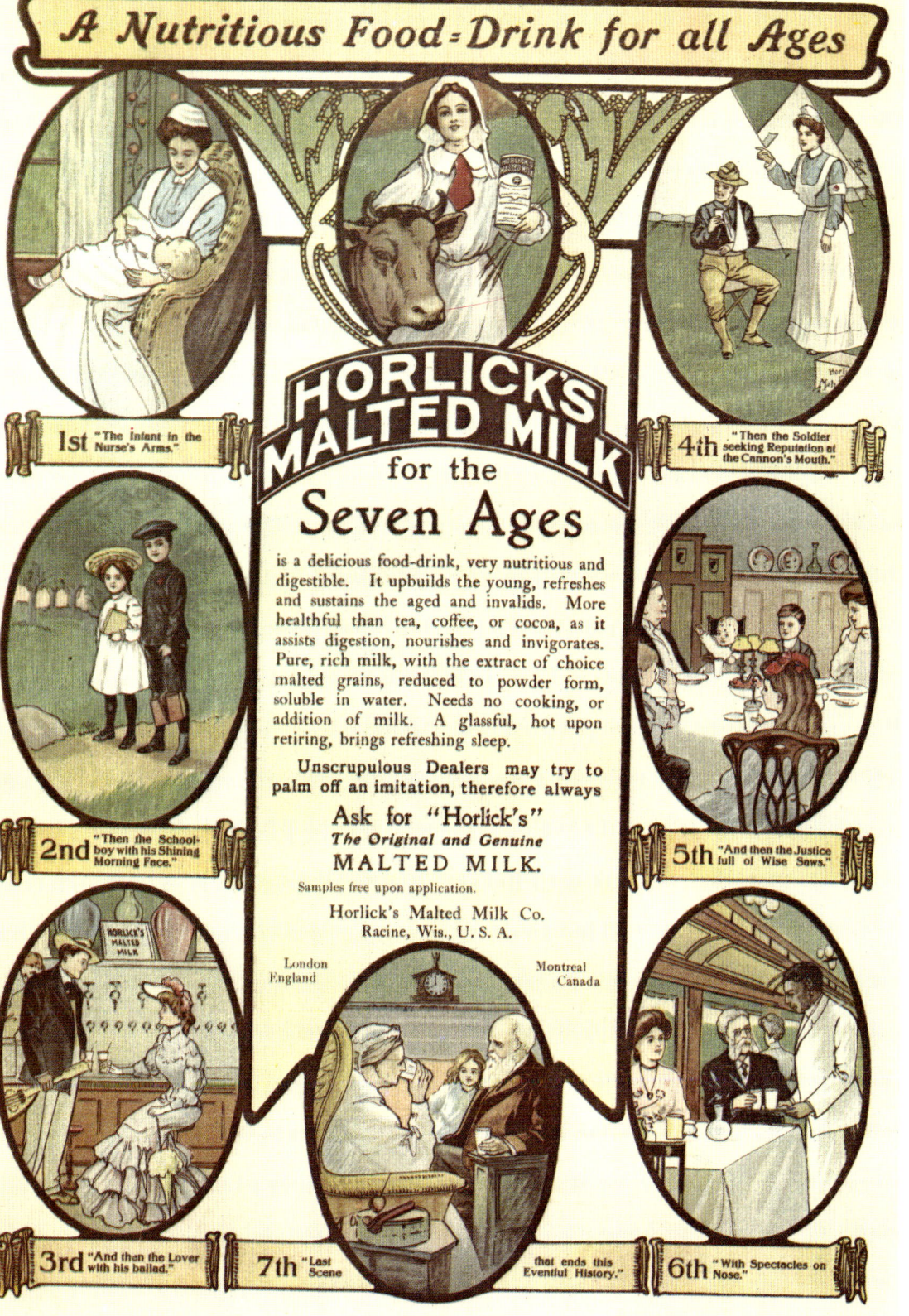

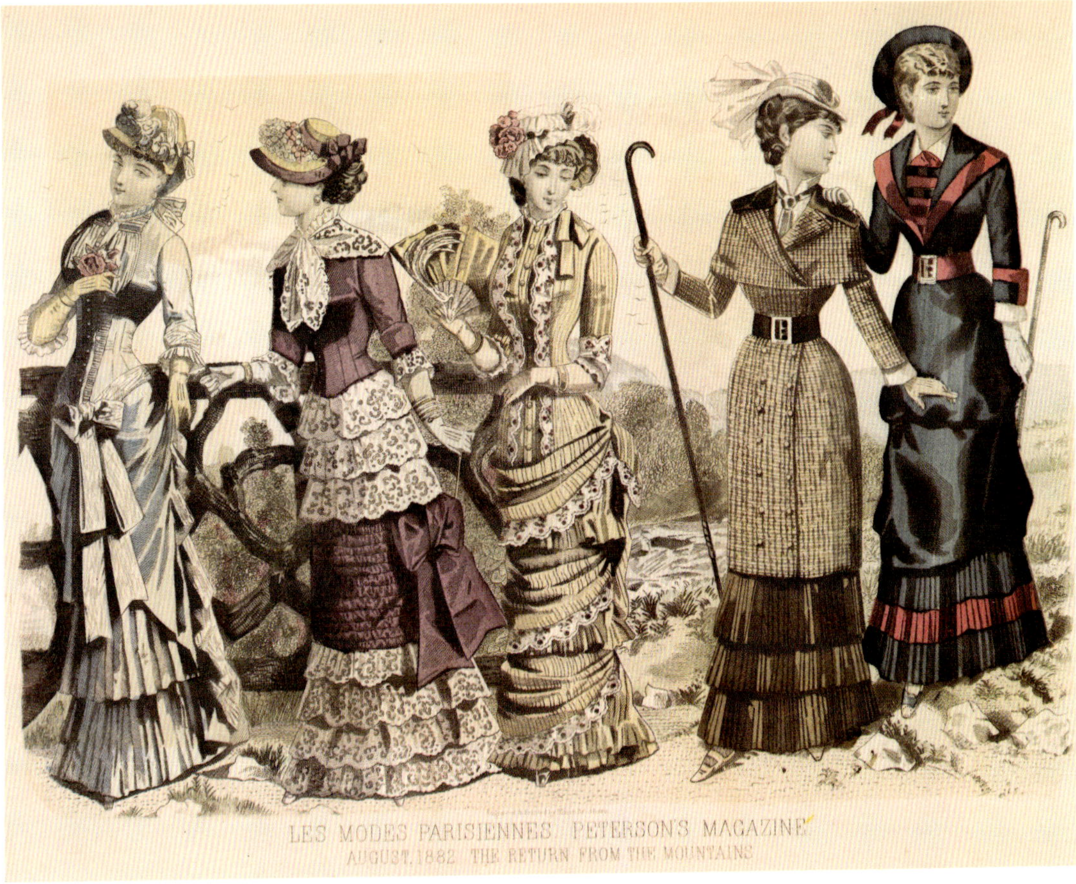

LES MODES PARISIENNES. PETERSON'S MAGAZINE.
AUGUST, 1882. THE RETURN FROM THE MOUNTAINS.

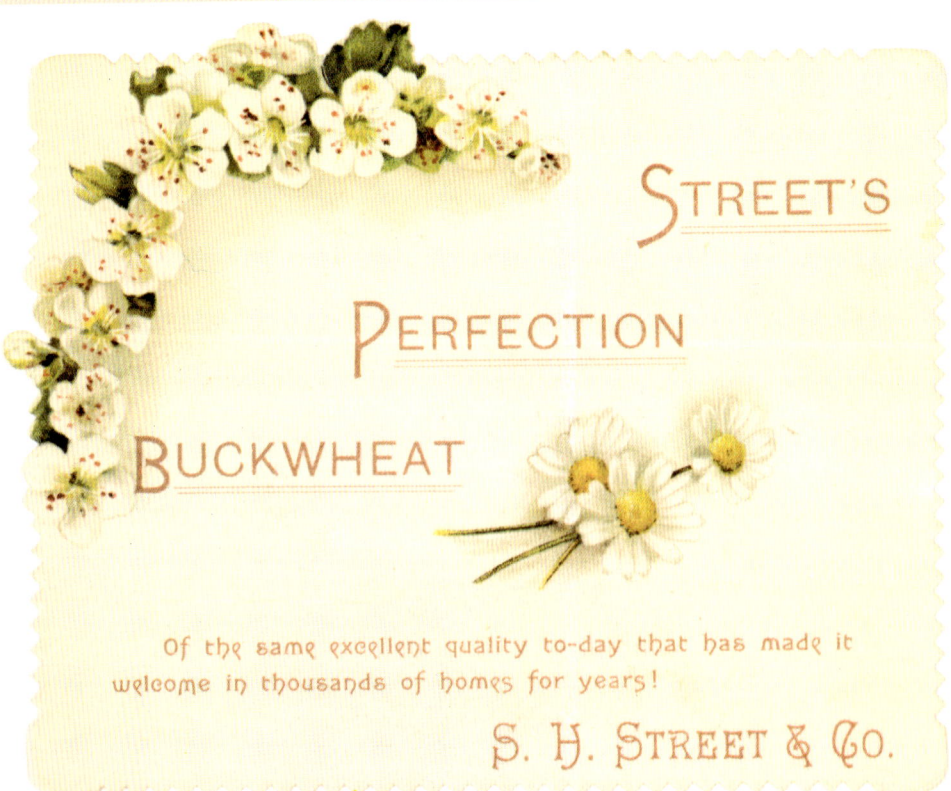

STREET'S

PERFECTION

BUCKWHEAT

Of the same excellent quality to-day that has made it welcome in thousands of homes for years!

S. H. Street & Co.

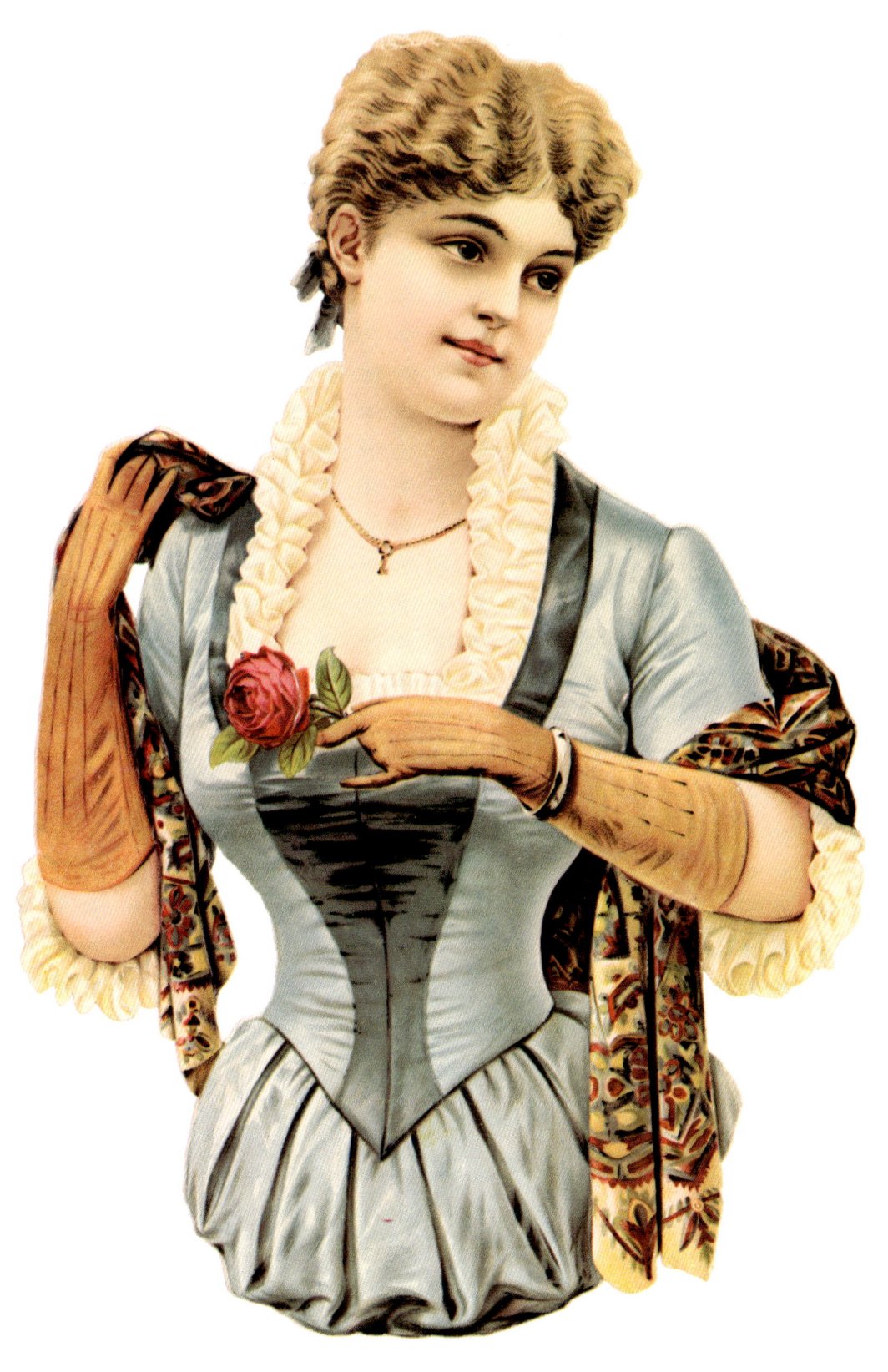

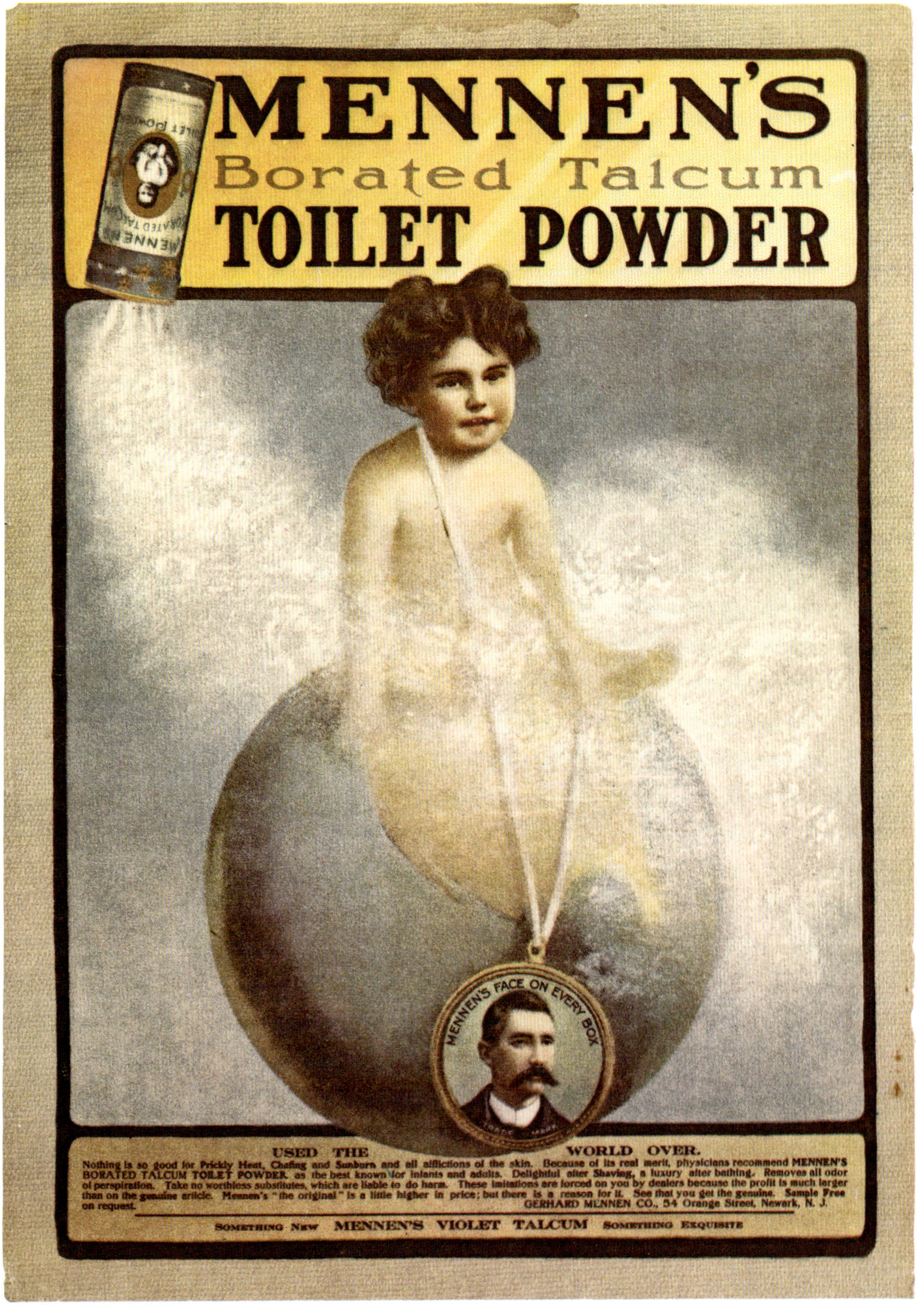

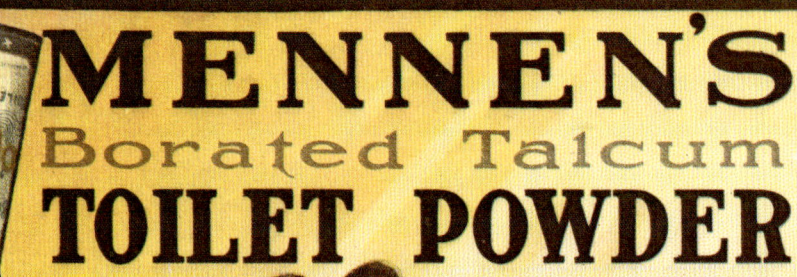

MENNEN'S
Borated Talcum
TOILET POWDER
MENNEN'S FACE ON EVERY BOX
USED THE WORLD OVER.
Nothing is so good for Prickly Heat, Chafing and Sunburn and all afflictions of the skin. Because of its real merit, physicians recommend MENNEN'S BORATED TALCUM TOILET POWDER as the best known for infants and adults. Delightful after Shaving, a luxury after bathing. Removes all odor of perspiration. Take no worthless substitutes, which are liable to do harm. These imitations are forced on you by dealers because the profit is much larger than on the genuine article. Mennen's "the original" is a little higher in price; but there is a reason for it. See that you get the genuine. Sample Free on request.
GERHARD MENNEN CO., 54 Orange Street, Newark, N. J.
SOMETHING NEW MENNEN'S VIOLET TALCUM SOMETHING EXQUISITE

Are You Fat?

Kellogg's Obesity Food Will Reduce Your Weight to Normal, Free You From Suffering and Turn Your Fat Into Muscle.

It Has Done This For Many Others Who Testify to Its Efficacy—Trial Package Free.

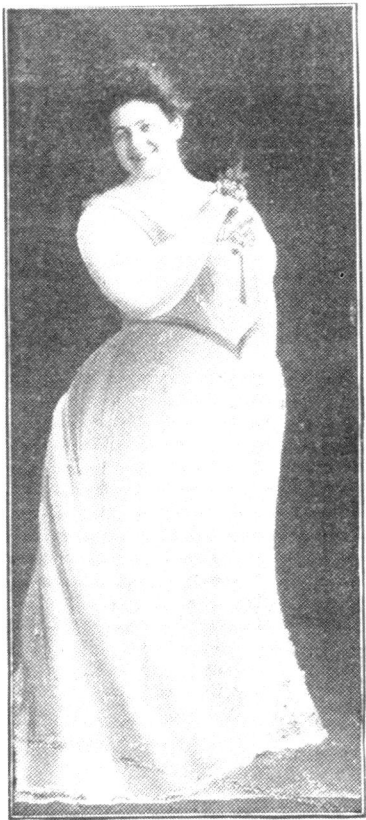 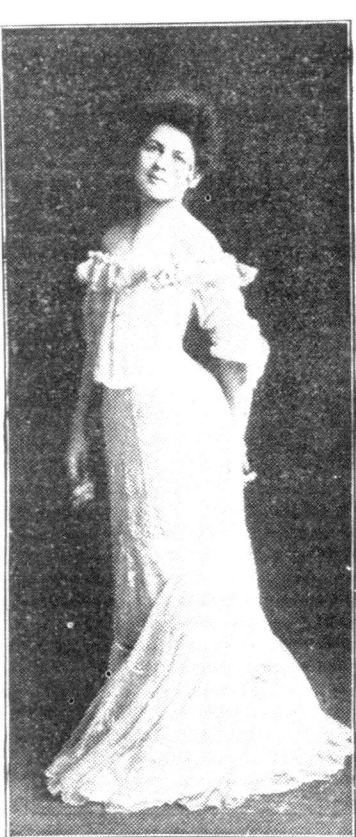

The Above Illustration Shows the Remarkable Effects of This Wonderful Obesity Food—What It Has Done For Others It Will Do For You.

Don't be fat. It is an abnormal and diseased condition of the body. Nutriment that should have built up bone and muscle for you has made fat instead.

Excess fat is attended by many dangers. The heart, stomach, liver and kidneys become seriously affected; breathing is made difficult and often, though seemingly well, the fat person is in grave danger.

Don't starve yourself. You will only become weakened and aggravate your condition without losing flesh.

There is a sure way and a safe way. Hundreds of reputable people testify to what Kellogg's Obesity Food has done for them. It has turned their fat into muscle. They submit their photographs as corroborative evidence. Can you doubt such proof?

Don't be fat. Write to me to-day and I will send you free, a trial package, postpaid, in plain wrapper.

One happy woman, Mrs. Etta Hamerick, 230 Fischer Ave., Detroit, Mich., says: "I have just finished the seven weeks' treatment of your Obesity Food, and must say that it is one of the most wonderful treatments that I have ever seen or heard of. It has simply converted me into a new woman. I have lost in weight eighty-three pounds in three months. My health is in every way improved, and I am no longer bothered with that smothered feeling which I used to have after the slightest exertion.

"I am sure that your treatment deserves all and even more than you claim for it. Never saw anything like it.

"You can refer anyone to me, and I will be glad to recommend your method, as I am ready and anxious to aid you, as well as all sufferers from surplus flesh."

Send your name and address—no money—to-day to F. J. Kellogg, 1968 Kellogg Bldg., Battle Creek, Mich., and receive the trial package in plain wrapper free by return mail.

The colonials were much more concerned with getting rid of freckles than we seem to be today, judging from the number of freckle removers in the old beauty books.

To Remove Freckles: Grate a fresh horse-radish root very fine, cover with fresh buttermilk, and let stand overnight. Strain through cheese cloth, and wash the face morning and night with the resulting liquor.

Or squeeze the juice of a lemon into half a tumbler of water, and use two or three times daily as a face wash.

Or dissolve in lemon juice as much sugar as it will hold, and apply with a soft brush frequently until the freckles disappear.

Or mix two ounces of lemon juice with one dram of confectioner's sugar or powdered rock candy and ½ dram of powdered borax. Let stand for four or five days, shaking occasionally, and apply with a soft camel's-hair brush two or three times a day.

(*Household Discoveries*, 1872)

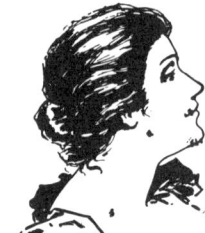

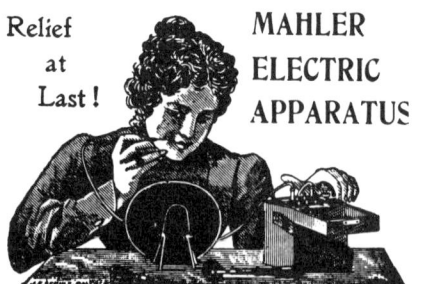

Household Tips

The colonials depended on candles for most of their artificial illumination and various bits of advice on the care and use of candles abound in all the old publications. This little gem helps avoid that unpleasant smell every time you extinguish one.

> TO BLOW OUT A CANDLE: Hold the candle higher than the mouth and blow it out by an upward instead of a downward air current. This will prevent the wick from smouldering.
>
> (*Allan's New England Almanack,* 1840)

I'm forever buying decanters and old bottles at auctions and tag sales, and before I found this method of cleaning them I had a lot of dirty bottles. I've found that chopped potatoes work on all but the filthiest specimens, and eggshells work when the potatoes fail.

> TO CLEAN BOTTLES: Various substances and a number of ingenious methods are employed to clean water bottles, wine decanters, milk bottles, and medicine bottles, the inside of which cannot be reached by ordinary methods. Among these are heavy articles such as tacks and shot, or lighter ones, as crushed eggshells, raw potatoes chopped fine, bits of cloth or paper to dislodge dirt and for mechanical cleansing. Also lye and various acids, as lemon juice, sour milk, and dilute hydrochloric acid.

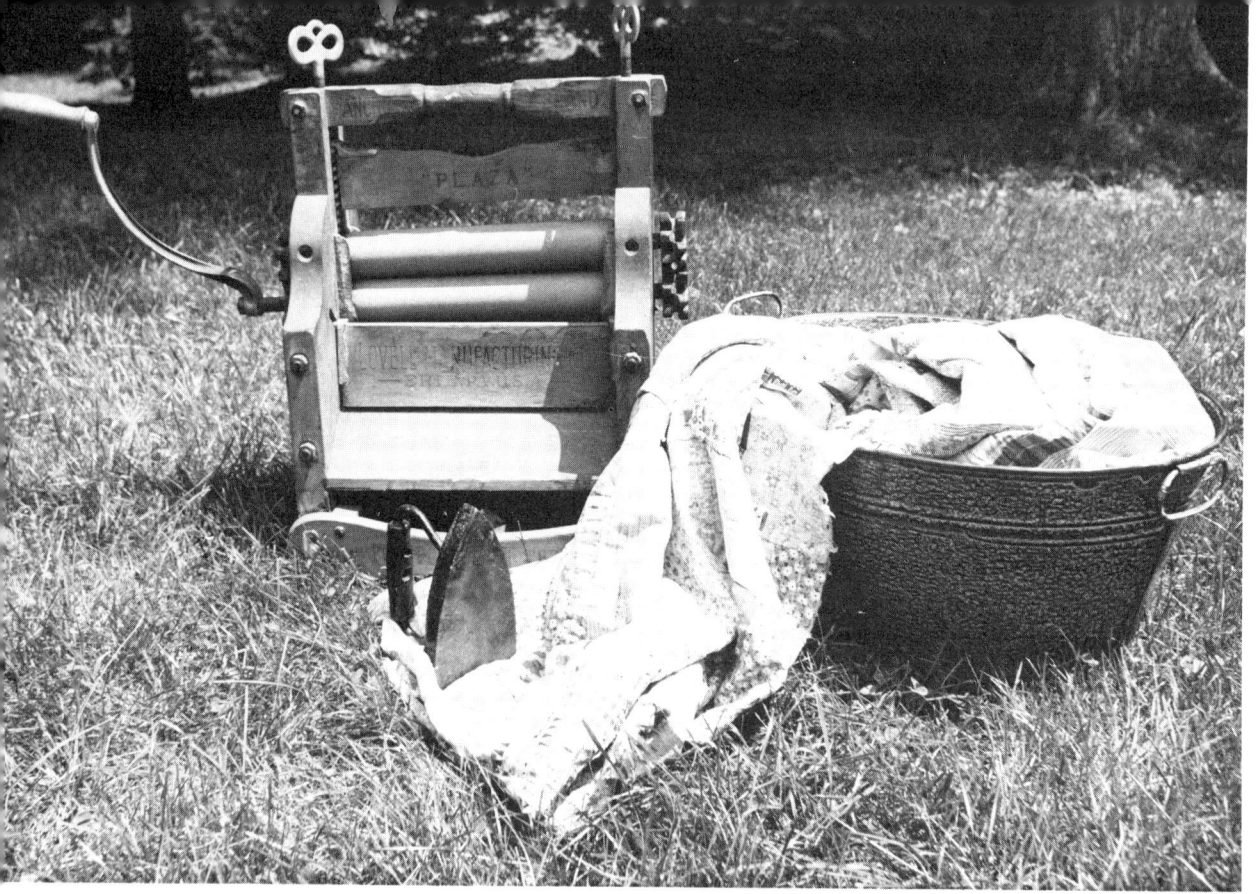

For coarse and heavy articles, like glass milk bottles and fruit jars, use a handful of common shot or carpet tacks. Fill the jar or bottle half-full of soapsuds, add the tacks or shot, and shake well. If tacks are used their sharp edges will scrape off the dirt, but will also scratch the bottle. Hence they are not suitable for wine or vinegar cruets, whether plain or cut glass. If shot is used care must be taken that none of them are suffered to remain in the cruets, or in bottles to contain any acid, as the action of acid upon lead produces deadly poison.

Or use one tablespoonful of crushed eggs in the same manner. If the bottle is greasy wash with warm water and a little soda, or run a raw potato through the meat chopper, put it in a bottle of warm water and shake until clean. This is one of the most effective cleansers known.

(*Household Advice,* 1855)

The next most common problem with old bottles with ground glass stoppers is that they often stick and are almost impossible to remove. This next bit of advice may seem obvious to some, but I've included it because it's so comprehensive. However, I still have some bottles which refuse to open, so if *you* have any suggestions....

GLASS STOPPERS: The glass stoppers of decanters and carafes and other bottles sometimes stick and are difficult to remove. To remove a stopper that sticks, first apply a few drops of olive or other oil to the neck of the stopper, and let stand a few minutes to soak in between the stopper and the neck of the bottle. If this does not loosen the stopper, apply heat to the neck of the bottle on the outside. It is a well-known fact that heat expands all substances, and if applied to the outside, the neck of the bottle will expand before the stopper does, and the stopper will become loosened. The best method for warming the bottle is to dip a rag in as hot water as the hands will bear and wrap it about the neck of the bottle. This must not be done, however, when the bottle is very cold, as it may be cracked by expanding too suddenly.

(*Household Advice*, 1855)

Just in case you're afflicted with yellowed piano keys....

TO KEEP IVORY PIANO KEYS WHITE: Keep the keys white by rubbing with a soft cloth wet with alcohol or cologne water. Expose the keys to sunshine on bright, sunny days to bleach them. If the keys seem brittle and cracked, rub them gently with a scrap of cotton wool moistened with olive oil.

(*Ballou's Magazine*, 1858)

I wouldn't use the following method on an Old Master, but if you have some paintings that simply aren't worth the cost of a professional cleaning this is a very effective and relatively safe procedure.

TO CLEAN OIL PAINTINGS: To clean an oil painting, wash the surface with clear warm water, using a soft flannel cloth or fine sponge, let dry, and rub gently with a soft flannel cloth moistened with pure olive oil. The water softens the accumulated dirt, smoke, and dust, and the oil assists in wiping it away.

Or wash with milk diluted with warm water, and dry without rinsing.

Or cut a potatoe in half and rub gently with the fresh surface, slicing off the soiled portions, until the whole is cleansed.

(*Success Magazine*, 1870)

This next gem is a real money-saver for those of you who have old pendulum clocks; this advice should save you more than a few visits to the watchmaker.

TO CLEAN CLOCKS: To clean a clock, saturate a cloth or pad of cotton with kerosene oil and lay it inside on a small dish that will prevent the woodwork from becoming saturated. As it evaporates, the fumes will loosen any foreign substance on the wheels of the clock and cause it to drop. Repeat as often as necessary—the fumes also tend to lubricate the works.

To OIL CLOCKS: Use only the purest olive oil and apply by means of a matchstick.

(*Household Advice*, 1850)

If you happen to have any carbon steel cutlery, this is a real time-saver!

To KEEP STEEL KNIVES FROM RUSTING: Keep in the pantry a deep box or crock containing fine, dry, sand and plunge the blades into this when not in use. This will prevent rust.

(*Farmer's Almanack*, 1830)

Ever struggled with a wax encrusted candlestick, scraping and cursing in a futile attempt to remove the tenacious goo? Well, here's a very old and very effective solution.

To CLEAN SILVER, METAL AND PORCELAIN CANDLESTICKS: To clean candlesticks, dip them in boiling water to remove grease and melted wax, and afterwards clean and polish them according to the material they are made of. Do not attempt to scratch off the wax or grease with a knife or melt it off with dry heat, especially if they are plated, as the plated-ware is often based on a composition which will be injured by this type of heating.

(*Peterson's National Ladies Magazine*, 1860)

This liquid will clean off the worst tarnish without injuring the silver.

To BOIL TARNISHED SILVER: If the silver is much tarnished, boil for five minutes in water containing a mixture of equal parts of cream of tartar, common salt, and alum, using one teaspoonful of each to one pint of water.

(*Household Advice*, 1855)

The last time I sent a small Oriental carpet to the rug cleaners I was amazed at how expensive it's become to have a rug cleaned. Commercial rug cleaning preparations are excellent for carpets with fast colors, but if you have an old Oriental you're not sure of, these following methods are very good, but preferably do your cleaning out of doors on a warm day, as kerosene is flammable.

To FRESHEN CARPETS: Before sweeping, scatter dry salt over the carpet. It brightens the colours and checks the ravages of moths. Or slightly moisten salt with kerosene. Sprinkle the carpet and sweep thoroughly. The dust will not rise, but will be thoroughly taken up by the mixture. The kerosene will leave no greasy effect, the odour will soon pass off, and the carpet will be wonderfully freshened. Corn meal may be substituted for the salt.

(*Household Advice,* 1874)

Several years ago a large mail-order company advertised a "miracle roach powder" which turned out to be nothing more than borax. Well, borax *is* a miracle roach powder—inexpensive, nonpoisonous, odorless, and *very* effective. And doesn't "Croton Bug" sound much better than "Roach"?

> To Exterminate Cockroaches also Known as the Croton Bug: Mix equal quantities of grated sweet chocolate and powdered borax, or equal quantities of powdered sugar and powdered borax, and spread freely on shelves where cockroaches run, or spread on slightly moistened bread.
>
> Or mix in a saucer one part of plaster of Paris and three parts of flour, and place in their runways. Place nearby another saucer containing pure water. Lay thin pieces of cardboard from one to the other as bridges and float on the water bits of thin board touching the margin. The cockroaches eat the flour and plaster of Paris, become thirsty, and drink. The plaster then sets and kills them. This is an Austrian method. It is simple, safe, and said to be very effective.
>
> But of all of the above, powdered borax, with or without flour, and powdered sugar, or both, is perhaps the safest and most useful remedy. It may be dusted freely on shelves, sinks, and kitchen floors, and also forced by means of a bellows, into cracks and crevices, about floors, baseboards, cupboards, sinks, et cetera. It is cheap and harmless to children and household pets, and is far superior to any so-called "cockroach powder" upon the market.

(*Household Advice,* 1875)

This method of cleaning wallpaper was in use before the era of plastic-coated and washable wallpapers, but if you happen to have any walls covered with good old-fashioned paper, this is a very effective way to get off the dirt.

We heard of an old gentleman, who was describing the scenes of the Revolutionary War, tell a story of some of the gun powder which was used in those days, which shows that he thought it not the best. He said a barrel of it happened to take fire one day, and *burnt half up before they could put it out!*

(*The American Domestic Cook Book,* 1868)

To Clean Wallpaper: Brush down the walls with a hairbrush or dustcloth, then cut a loaf of yeastbread two or three days old once vertically through the middle, and again crosswise. Hold these pieces by the crust and rub the wall downward with long, light strokes. Do not rub across the paper, or rub harder than necessary.
(*Ballou's Magazine,* 1865)

This is my all-time favorite household receipt. I've never tried it, but just the knowledge that someone thought up a way to gild live goldfish fills me with a feeling akin to a heady drunkenness!

To Gild Live Goldfish: Smear the inside of an earthen bowl with white pitch, warm it gently, and scatter pulverized amber over the pitch. Remove from the fire, add three pounds of oleum lini and one pound of oleum terebinth mixed together. Cover and boil for one hour with gentle heat. Mix with powdered pumice stone to the consistency of paint. Take a live fish from the water, dry it by means of a cloth, and apply this paint with a brush. Immediately spread gold leaf over it, and rub dry with a soft cloth. Return the fish to the water. The longer this varnish is under the water the harder it grows, and does the fish no harm.
(*Household Discoveries,* 1850)

First you have to catch the rat!

To Drive Away Rats: Coal tar mixed with sand to the consistency of thick mortar, is an effectual stopper to ratholes. Or, rats may be driven off by catching one, soaking him in coal tar, and letting him run.
(*Dr. Herrick's American Domestic Receipt Book,* 1868)

In 1850, love letters came under the heading "Receipts For The Household."

Love Letters: For a love letter, good paper is indispensable. When it can be procured, that of a costly quality, gold-edged, perfumed, or ornamented in the French style, may be properly used. The letter

No teacher who regards his duties in the light of reason and religion, can look upon them as repulsive, or monotonous, or irksome. The angel that unlocks the gates of heaven, might as well become weary of his service, though with every opening door, a new spirit is ushered into the mansions of bliss.
(*Farmer's Almanack,* 1840)

should be carefully enveloped, and nicely sealed with a fancy wafer—not a common one of course, where any other can be had; or what is better, plain or fancy sealing wax. As all persons are more or less governed by first impressions and externals, the whole affair should be as neat as possible.

(*Married Ladies' Indispensable Companion and Family Physician,* 1850)

Through the years I've come across many household tips that I've remembered, but no longer remember where I found them. The following are a few that are bound to be useful to you sooner or later.

TO LUBRICATE KITCHEN MACHINERY: Glycerin makes an excellent lubricant for egg beaters or other kitchen utensils that have moving parts.

TO WHITEN LACES: To whiten discolored laces, wash them in sour milk.

TO REMOVE BURNED ON STARCH FROM YOUR IRON: Sprinkle salt on a piece of brown paper and slide the iron back and forth several times. Then polish with powdered pumice (or silver polish) until the roughness and stain are removed.

TO MAKE BROOMS LAST LONGER: Dip a new broom in hot salt water before using. This will toughen the bristles and make them less likely to break.

Here's a delicious way to preserve fruit if you have access to a large quantity of honey. Of course, you can always make a small batch—enough to fill a pint canning jar is an ideal amount to experiment with.

TO KEEP PLUMS AND PEACHES RIPE THROUGHOUT THE YEAR: Beat up well together honey and spring water, equal amounts, put freshly gathered fruit into an earthen vessel and pour this over, and cover close. Wash them when wanted for use.

(*Mrs. Abell's Receipts,* 1850)

This method is a whole lot easier to use than the wet tissue paper and aluminum foil method, and the results are much better.

TO TRANSPORT FLOWERS FRESH: Place them in a wide-mouthed bottle, with only a small aperture for the admission of air. The exhalation of the leaves is a moisture that refreshes and sustains them.

(*Household Advice,* 1860)

Since gardening was a subject cookbooks and almanacs invariably dealt with, I've included this rather lengthy piece on "Things To Be

Remembered In The Cultivation of Flowers," especially for those of you who have just taken up gardening as a pastime and are in need of some general rules and pointers.

THINGS TO BE REMEMBERED IN THE CULTIVATION OF FLOWERS: Sun and air, are as important to flowers as the lungs and heart to man. Clay soil mixed with ashes will make a good mould. The black soil is the richest, and should be dug in the fall, and a foot renewed once in three years.

Stones and weeds should be often removed, they are like blemishes on the face of beauty. Almost every plant loves sand, it is especially good for bulbs, pinks, carnations, hyacinths, auriculas, &c; at least one-third should be sand.

No flower garden should be without monthly roses and pinks. They will reward labour by ceaseless bloom, are hardy and easily cultivated. By a covering of straw in the fall, they will live out, or they may be kept in the cellar, or blossom in the parlour as a winter solace.

A light spade, two rakes, one with very fine teeth, the other a size larger, for cleaning the walks, and for raking large stones from the garden borders; a light fork for taking up bulbous or delicate roots, a watering pot, a hoe, and a trowel, pruning knife, and shears, are the tools for flower gardening. A pair of India rubbers will enable a lady to indulge her passion for flowers at all seasons, without risk of life or health in fair weather, and will operate beneficially on the mind and body. Who would of choice live without flowers?

Sun-flowers and Holly-hocks look best as a screen to some unsightly object, or in the background in clumps of three and three, but not in connection with the more delicate and choicer flowers. Plant Holly-hocks in September or October, as a late flower they are invaluable.

Annuals are those flowers which are raised from seed in the spring, and die in autumn.

Biennials are those produced by seed, bloom the second year, remain two years in perfection, and then gradually dwindle away and die. Some sorts will be improved and perpetuated by offsets, slips, and cuttings of the tops. Wall flowers, Sweet Williams, Rockets, and Carnations will become double, by slips of the small tops, shoots, layers, and pipings.

Perennials are those flowers which continue many years, and are propagated by root-offsets, suckers, parting roots, &c.

Flowers should be so arranged as to have a succession of them through the season on the same beds. Decaying flowers, should be cheered by the bloom of youth and beauty.

Those that bloom in March or April of the common kind are,

Valuable Hints to Mothers.

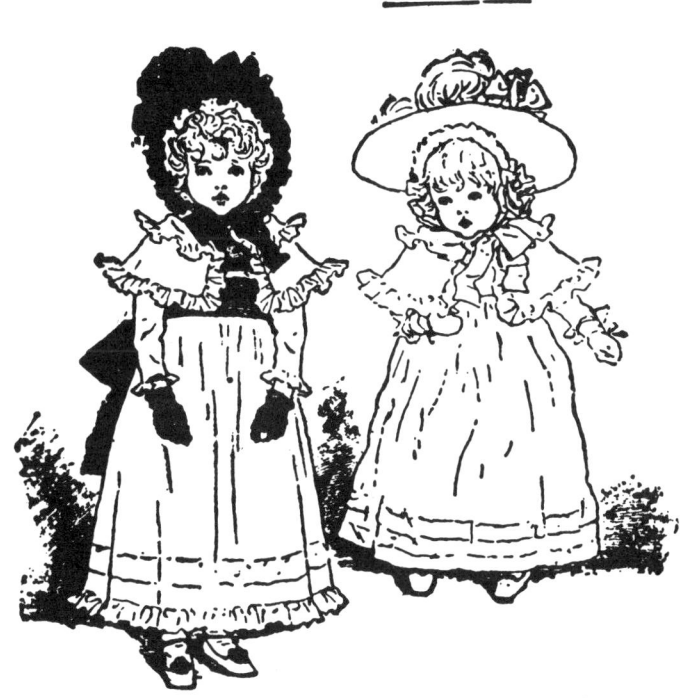

Never let a child sob itself to sleep.

Onions in any form are good for children.

When a child refuses to eat let him have his own way.

A little borax in baby's bath water is good for his skin.

Oil of cloves will often cure an aching tooth.

Mustard plasters made with the white of egg do not blister.

Cats carry sore throats and diphtheria from house to house.

A hair mattress is better than a feather bed.

To ensure pure water for drinking purposes boil it.

If a child's clothes catch fire, instantly roll him on the floor.

Daffodils, Crocuses, Jonquils, Hyacinths, Polyantuses, Single Primroses which are very beautiful; Yellow Gilliflower, Narcissus, Liverwort, Anemones, Pansies, Daisies, Iris, Crown Imperial, Spring Cyclamens, Forward Bear's Ears, March Violets.

May—Day Lilies, Lily of the Valley, Mountain Pinks, Italian Spiderwort, Poet's Pinks, Peonies, Columbines, Double Jacea, a sort of Lychnis; Orange Lilies, Bastard Dittany, Ranunculuses, Tulips, Asphodels, Cyanususes, &c.

June—Snap-dragons, Tuberoses, Larkspurs, Monkshoods, Pinks, Foxgloves, Candytufts, Poppies, Roses of all kinds, the month of Roses!

July—Most of the June flowers, except Roses, Jessamine, Bell Flowers, Dittanies, Amaranthuses, Hellebore, Double Marigolds, Lilies of all kinds, Belvideres, Tri-colours, Sea-hollies, Spanish Broom, &c.

August—Most of those of July, Marvels of Peru, Starwort, White Bell Flower, Indian Narcissus, Passion Flower, Evening Primrose, &c.

September—Most of those of July, Amaryllis, Narcissus of Portugal, Indian Roses, Autumnal Crocus, Carnations, Colchicums, Petunias, &c.

October—The same, with China Asters, Autumn Crocus, Violets. Monthly Roses and Pinks every month.

(*The Mother's Book Of Daily Duties,* 1855)

Well, modern meteorologists may say these are just a collection of old wives tales, but I've found these methods just as accurate as the 11 O'Clock News...

A FEW INDICATIONS OF WEATHER: Rule 1st. If the sun rise red and fiery you may expect wind and rain; if cloudy, and the clouds soon decrease, certain fair weather; if, in the morning, some parts of the sky appear green between the clouds, while the sky is blue above, stormy weather is not far off.

2nd. Clouds small, strewed with dapple grey, with a North Wind bring fair weather for two or three days; clouds that look like large rocks portend large showers; on the other hand if large clouds decrease, it is proof of fair weather in summer or harvest time; if clouds rise with great white tops, and joined together with black on the lowest side, especially if two such clouds arise, make haste, rain is near.

3d. If mist arises in low grounds and soon vanishes, it is a token of fair weather; and if it rises high, or to the tops of hills, you may expect rain in a day or two; a general mist before the sun rises, near the full of the moon, brings rain in the end.

4th. Sudden rains do not last long. If it begins to rain an hour or two before sun rising, it is likely to rain all that day, except the rainbow be seen before it begins to rain.

5th. When at night you hear the sound of bells, water, beasts, or any other noise unassisted by the wind in that direction it is inclined to rain. The sinking of rivers, indicate that much rain will follow; the reverse after rain denotes dry weather.

If the earth or moist place emit a strong smell, rain follows. Dews lying long in the morning, signify fair weather; small dews and soon vanishing, rain.

If the colours of the Rainbow tend more to red than any other colour, wind follows; if green or blue, then rain.

Generally a moist and cool summer portends a hard winter. A hot and dry summer and autumn, especially if the heat and drought extend far into September, portend an open beginning for winter, and cold latter part of it, and beginning of Spring.

A warm, open winter, portends a hot and dry summer, for the vapours disperse in the winter showers, whereas, cold and frost keep them in, and convey them to spring and summer.

(*Allan's Almanack,* 1830)

ALARMING EFFECT OF TOBACCO SMOKE: A post-mortem examination recently made on a young man who had died during the night, the physician pronounced he had died of congestion of the brain, caused by the respiration of tobacco smoke, during sleep.

(*Allan's Almanack,* 1835)

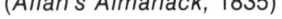

Useful Hint: The difference between rising every morning at six and at eight, in the course of forty years (supposing a man to go to bed at the same time he otherwise would) amounts to 20,000 hours, or three years, 121 days and 16 hours, which will afford eight hours a day for exactly ten years; so that it is the same as if ten years of life were added, in which we could commend eight hours every day for the cultivation of our minds, and the dispatch of our beliefs.

(*Beer's Almanac,* 1800)

An Odd & An End

A View of Women's Lib circa 1855

A truly accomplished woman is one who turns her time to the best account, either imparting or receiving instruction, or promoting the welfare and comfort of those around her, in domestic and social life.

Female industry enobles and dignifies the highest station, and the lowest is beautified by its presence. It is an amaranthine flower that blooms in perpetual beauty when the more frail flowers of life have all perished.

In contemplating a woman who is skilled in the various arts of life, who is thoroughly accomplished and complete in her character, so constituted by her own industry and intelligence, we feel there is something that will last and live when her fine complexion has lost its rose tint, and the eye its brilliant glow, and the soft hair its colour and silken lustre.

The weak and silly idea that idleness and ignorance constitute a lady, is fast passing away! Woman's mission, for this age, is beginning to be felt and understood, and we hope the time is not far distant when occupation and effort will take the place of discontent—

ennui—and debility—which characterizes too many of the frail daughters of our land.

What noble examples have we in the past—Queens regulated their own household matters, and used their jewelled and delicate hands in useful occupation.

Ladies of nobility and rank, whose names have been considered worthy of an honourable rememberance, were not only good housekeepers, but they established schools and churches, and were themselves active in providing for the industry and necessities of the poor. And not only this, but they became distinguished in literature, and are bright stars in the horizon of past ages.

What a model of industry was Hannah More. Although often a sufferer, yet what a monument of worth and industrious effort is her beautiful and noble character. It is garlanded too, with such blossoms as never fade, or grow dim with age or time.

It is only by the dint of application and effort that great results are ever accomplished. Unless there is some habit formed, and something undertaken, life will pass away with but the trifles of the hour, and no trace will be left that an *active* human being has ever lived!

Look at our mothers in their bright sunny days of girlhood. They were no idlers! Their faces gleamed with health and beauty; ambition and energy sent the true-life carmine to the cheek and the brightest lustre to the eye.

Imported goods were forbidden by law, and their originality and invention were put to the test. There could be no embroidery until their hands had first combed, spun and dyed the cruels, made the canvass, and saved time, by a greater effort in common duties, to blend their beautiful shades and colours.

Feminine taste was not destroyed by the pressure of the times, but would occasionally shine out to adorn its rigours.

Fathers and brothers had gone at their country's call, yielding all selfish motives to the public good, obliged to leave the stern duties of the farm and all masculine employments in the hands of wives and daughters, old men and boys. This was the case with the families of the highest officers in the armies of the Revolution. What an accumulated weight this brought upon them—but they shrunk not aghast at the burden! Their fair hands were often on the rake or the hoe, and their beautiful round arms encircled the harvests while they

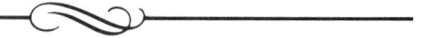

Men are of two sorts: those who think, and those who amuse themselves.

(*Connecticut Pocket Almanack*, 1802)

both aided and superintended every department in the field and the house.

The more there was to be done, the greater was the power to accomplish; and the wheel and the loom only had an increased momentum, and sung a merrier tune, while the roses on the cheeks and lips blossomed into deeper colour.

They wrought from the flax delicate and rich linen laces, beautiful lawns, and various kinds of fabrics beside those for common and necessary use.

Genius and talent were displayed in a great variety of ways, and heroines were abundant.

The "Women of the Revolution," as sketched by Mrs. Ellet, is full of the heroism, energy and industry of the times; and if it awakens a new impulse in our own age, operating, of course, in different channels, she will not have laboured in vain.

There are a great variety of methods in which female talent and industry may find ample scope, and be turned to good account; and we have many fine illustrations of the capabilities of the sex at the present day.

We do not demand nor desire for woman what some of late are exerting themselves with so much eloquence to accomplish. Her "rights" we expect will be well cared for by those who are constituted by nature and religion her protectors.

Man should so construct our laws that her helplessness shall be protected, her property kept inviolate, and it will come back to him in four-fold blessings.

And when the great avenues, which bring wretchedness and poverty into her home to darken her existence and paralize her faculties, are closed up forever, her hopes will be crowned with fruition, and her heart filled with tearful joy, for then her industry will indeed be a beauty and an ornament to her household, and her toils shall not be drudgery performed with a poor broken heart, but with the noble sentiment that it is for those she loves.

Females of this age have not the same duties nor the same necessities as those of an earlier period. Everything is changed, both in the facilities and requisitions of labour. Yes, woman need not go out of her appropriate sphere for duties and high motives to perform them.

Why is a husband like a Mississippi steamboat? Because he never knows when he may get a blowing up.
(*The American Domestic Cook Book,* 1868)

Wealth releases many from the strong and exacting demand or late and early toil, but it should not release them from obligations and imperative duties. No woman of right moral feeling will appropriate her precious time to the silly strife of fashion, or the giddy round of pleasure, and be satisfied with merely passing her time in ease and personal gratification. She will feel there is something higher and nobler to live for, and she will employ her priceless hours in aiding forward and in divising plans for usefullness, for with the means, she has the power to accomplish great and useful results.

There is enough in every sphere of life, and in every station, for the full and perfect development of female mind and character. There is no occasion for woman to feel that her sphere is narrow and unimportant.

A thorough and right education would open her eyes to the magnitude of her duties, and the strength of intellect that is requisite to perform those duties with honour and credit, with comfort and ease, and at the same time she would not shrink from them, preferring indolence and inactivity to a life well spent.

Beside the home occupations, from which very few are entirely exempt, society has claims upon her, and its conditions in her own immediate circle will be the truest index to what she has done, and what influence she has exerted.

Benevolence—where it can expect to find an abode if not in the heart of a woman, warm with every generous impulse and kindly feeling. Its work she must do, or the miserable and poor and destitute must suffer and mourn in anguish.

If she witholds her influence from the objects that will benefit society, and bring blessings into her midst, angels may well mourn, and weep, if tears can fall from their sinless eyes.

How much has been done by her activity and efforts, while at the same time no domestic obligation has been lightly esteemed or overlooked. It often requires the nicest calculation and adjustment of time, it may have prevented her enjoying many an hour of ease, but, after all, she has the higher satisfaction that "she has done what she could."

Female education is never completed—woman is ever a learner—she is not debarred the privilege of any acquisition which her capabilities or inclination choose for herself. If she has the time the sources are ample and overflowing with mental wealth, as much at her disposal and use as she can desire, and why should she not fill her mind with its gems, and then scatter in profusion such gathered treasure?

Together with all useful occupations, and every domestic

accomplishment, let her so economize time that she may also acquire and add every embellishment.

Let every gift which God has so freely bestowed be cultivated to its highest extent.

Let her be an artist, if that power has been given her, and not think she is out of her sphere, or misimproving in her time. The art of drawing should be one of the essentials of female education. Its benefits are too numerous and important to be overlooked or lightly esteemed. It improves the judgment, elevates the taste, and gives much correctness to the eye that all other departments of skill will own its influence and acknowledge its utility.

Be not drones in the hive of life, but go out and find honey, and bring it yourself from every flower.

Music, embroidery, artificial flower-work, need not infringe upon a single duty, and what home is not more beautiful for all such embellishments, produced by the skill of busy fingers and well-improved time.

How useful is woman in the capacity of teacher. Here she has full scope for every acquirement, and room for the development and manifestation of all the virtues, and all the graces.

Her influence too in this position is immortal, transferred as it is to a mind destined to live forever.

As a mother her industry and powers need not languish for the want of appropriate occupation, for inquisitive childhood demands every question fully explained, and philosophical reasons given for all it sees or feels. She must be thoroughly furnished, or lose the respect of her child, and consequently her influence.

Her reading should be ample and judicious, not wasting time over that which will do no good.

The world should be better, happier, gentler for her having lived, while she should constantly remember that for every talent given for every hour wasted in idleness or folly "she must give account."

(*The Mother's Book Of Daily Duties*, 1855)

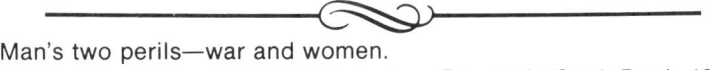

Man's two perils—war and women.
(*The American Domestic Cook Book*, 1868)

It is no great misfortune to oblige an ungrateful person; but an insupportable one to be under an obligation to a scoundrel.
(*Connecticut Pocket Almanac*, 1803)

Conversation

The object of conversation is to entertain and amuse. To be agreeable, you must learn to be a good listener. A man who monopolises a conversation is a *bore,* no matter how great his knowledge. Never get into a dispute. State your opinions, but do not argue them. Do not contradict, and, above all, never offend by correcting mistakes or inaccuracies of fact or expression.

Never lose temper—never notice a slight—never seem conscious of an affront, unless it is of a gross character.

You are not required to defend your friends in company, unless the conversation is addressed to you; but you may correct a statement of fact, if you know it to be wrong.

Never talk at people, by hints, slurs, innuendoes, and such mean devices. If you have anything to say, out with it. Nothing charms more than candor, when united with good breeding.

Do not call people by their names, in speaking to them. In speaking of your own children, never "Master" or "Miss" them—in speaking to other people of theirs, never neglect to do so.

It is very vulgar to talk in a loud tone, and indulge in hoarse laughs.

Be careful in speaking of subjects upon which you are not acquainted. Much is to be learned by confessing your ignorance—nothing can be by pretending to knowledge you do not possess.

Never tell long stories. Avoid all common slang phrases, and pet words.

Of all things, don't attempt to be too fine. Use good honest English—and common words for common things.

(*Married Ladies' Indispensable Companion and Family Physician,* 1850)

A young gentleman advertised in the papers for a wife, and received answers from eighteen-hundred husbands saying he could have theirs.

(*New England Almanac,* 1870)

It is more dishonorable to distrust a friend than it is to be deceived by him.

(*Astrological Calendar,* 1803)

Those who are themselves incapable of crimes are ever unsuspicious of others.

(*Beer's Almanac,* 1817)

The passions are the only orators that are always sure to persuade.
(Isaiah Thomas, *Junr's Almanac,* 1809)

Look at the catalog of criminals, the outcasts of society. In most cases they are grown up, ignorant and neglected children, the mind a blank or blot, and the heart foul with folly and corruption, which might have been, with proper care and culture, the fountain sending forth pure waters. Delays are dangerous. And what a multitude of such minds now surround round us, pleading through the gladsome eye of childhood, for care and education to save them from ruin. This is the field for the noblest Philanthropy. Who will plant the first flower?

(*The Mother's Book Of Daily Duties,* 1855)

Lord Falkland, the author of the play called The Marriage Night, was chose very young to sit in Parliament; and when he was first elected, some of the members opposed his admission, urging, that he had not sowed his wild oats; "Then," replied he, "it will be the best way to sow the remainder in the House, where there are so many geese to pick them up."

(*Strong's Astronomical Diary,* 1804)

Whatever real merit you have, other people will discover; and people always magnify their own discoveries as they lessen those of others.

(Isaiah Thomas, *Junr's Almanac,* 1810)

The reason why fools so often succeed in their plans is, that never distrusting themselves, they always persevere.

(*Allan's New England Almanack,* 1834)

Books are to the soul what the sun is to the earth: they enlighten it and qualify it for society.

(*Allan's New England Almanack,* 1801)

It must be learned early that the object of education is to form the character, rather than to inculcate knowledge. Everything which molds the disposition, gives direction to the taste and propensities, and decides which of the passions shall predominate, is the most important part in education.

(*The Family Almanack,* 1840)

Glossary of Terms & Measures

ALE: Colonial ale was much darker and stronger than today's ale. An authentic substitute would be a strong dark stout such as Guinness stout, or a strong dark German beer.

ALLSPICE: A spice native to the West Indies. The dried berry has an anesthetic effect when used in ointments. The dried berry is also used in cooking and preserving.

ALMOND MEAL: Sweet almonds which have been ground into a fine meal. Used in cosmetics and as a facial scrub.

ALUM: Used as an astringent in cosmetics and medicines. Available at your drugstore.

ANGELICA: An aromatic herb used in confectionery, perfumery, and to flavor liquors.

APERIENT: A mild laxative.

AQUA VITAE: A strong liquor without flavor. A good replacement is 100-proof Vodka.

AROMATIC: An aromatic plant, drug, or compound.

ARROWROOT POWDER: The powdered root of the arrowroot

plant. Used as a thickening agent and as a substitute for talcum. Available at your grocery store in the spice section.

AVOCADO PEAR: An old term for avocado.

BAIN MARIE: The French term for a double-boiler.

BALM: Also called Melissa, Lemon Balm and Bee Balm. It is a member of the mint family with a distinctive flavor and fragrance of lemons. Used medicinally to relieve fevers and inflammations; used as a flavoring in beverages and cooking.

BALM OF GILEAD: Also called Balsam and Mecca Balsam. Used medicinally to ease respiratory problems and as a soothing lotion for skin inflammations.

BAY SALT: A type of salt which is very coarse. A good substitute is kosher salt, available in most supermarkets.

BEAR GREASE: Purified fat from bear meat. Available from Caswell-Massey.

BENJAMIN: See Benzoin.

BENZOIN: The fragrant gum produced by trees in the Near East. It is used as a fixative in potpourris and other fragrant concoctions; medicinally as an antiseptic and preservative. To prepare a tincture of benzoin follow the instructions under "Tincture."

BLACK BRAMBLE BERRIES: Blackberries.

BORAGE: An herb used in medicinal preparations to reduce fever and inflammation. It is also used as a garnish in some beverages.

BROWN SOAP: Old-fashioned kitchen soap which is still available in supermarkets under the brand names Kirkmans Borax and Octagon.

BURDOCK: An herb that is considered one of the best blood purifiers; used externally for insect bites and other skin inflammations.

CALAMUS: Also called Sweet-Flag. The root of this herb is used as a tonic and stimulant. Some use it to kill their desire for tobacco.

CAMOMILE: Used medicinally in lotions to firm the tissues, clear inflamed eyes, and ease weariness. It is also used as an excellent hair rinse for blondes and as a tea to induce sleep. Grown in the herb garden it is said to repel insects.

CAMPHOR: Also called Gum Camphor and Laurel Camphor. Obtained from the camphor tree which grows in Formosa. It is used as an insect repellent and medicinally as a salve and inhalent.

CANDY HEIGHT: A term used in old recipes for candy and sugar syrups. The modern equivalent on a candy thermometer is 250–266 degrees Fahrenheit.

CAPILLAIRE: A syrup made with sugar and water.

CARDAMON (also CARDAMUM): An aromatic spice consisting of the seeds of an herb. It is used as a flavoring and in purgatives and tonics.

CHERRY LAUREL: Common European evergreen shrub.

CHOREA: A nervous disorder marked by spasmodic movements and incoordination.

CINNAMON: Used as a flavoring in cooking and in any number of medicinal preparations. Oil of Cinnamon is called Oil of Cassia in Great Britain.

CLOVE: The bud of the flower from an evergreen common to Indonesia. They are mainly used as a flavoring and to impart their scent to fragrant concoctions. Medicinally, Oil of Clove is used as a local anesthetic and as a cure for vomiting. Clove is also used as an antiseptic.

COCOA BUTTER (also THEOBROMA): The by-product obtained in the manufacture of chocolate. It is used as an excellent skin moisturizer, and by women to lessen stretch marks after childbirth.

DAMASK ROSE: A very fragrant rose used by the colonials in potpourris and other rose preparations. It was the only rose they grew in their herb gardens.

DANDELION: The common "weed" in your lawn. The greens are much favored in salads, the flowers used to make wine, the white "milk" used to remove warts, the dried and roasted roots as a coffee substitute. These are sometimes referred to in old herbals as "Piss-A-Beds."

DECANT: To pour off a liquid that has been allowed to settle without disturbing the sediment that has settled out.

DECOCTION: A liquid preparation made by boiling an herb or fruit with water, usually one part of herb or fruit to fifteen or twenty parts of water, in a covered nonmetal container, for fifteen to twenty minutes.

DEMULCENT: A liquid taken to soothe inflamed mucous membranes and prevent further irritation.

DIAPHORETIC: A substance that increases or causes perspiration.

DIURETIC: A substance that increases the flow of urine, thereby cleansing the excretory system.

DROPSY: Edema.

DYSPEPSIA: Indigestion.

ELDERBERRIES: Used both medicinally and as food throughout the world. Both the berries and flowers are used in cosmetics. The colonials made a sweet wine from the berries.

ELIXIR: A sweet, aromatic preparation, generally about 25% alcohol, used as a vehicle for medicines to make them more palatable.

FILTRATE: To filter. I use Chemex coffee filters folded into a cone-shape, supported in the mouth of a canning jar.

FLAX: The plant from which linen is made. The seeds of the flax are used medicinally as a demulcent and emollient.

GLYCERIN: A by-product in soap making. It is sweet, thick and colorless, and is used as a sweetener in medicines and tonics and as a base for many cosmetics. Available at drugstores.

GOUT: A disease marked by painful inflammation of the joints.

GREEN TEA: Tea that hasn't been dried and processed in the same way as the tea we're accustomed to. Used in colonial times in punches. Available in specialty stores and Japanese markets.

GROUND RICE: Rice flour.

HARICOT BEANS: A variety of green stringbeans.

HELIOTROPE: A plant with fragrant flowers which when inhaled are said to soothe the nerves.

HOPS: The dried flowers are used in the manufacture of beer, and brewed into tea are used as a cure for insomnia, restlessness, and to reduce fever and pain. Sewn into a pillow they help to induce sleep. Available from Nichols Garden Nursery.

INFUSION: The extraction of the useful properties of a substance by steeping, usually in water, sometimes in alcohol.

JASMINE: A tropical flower related to the gardenia. Its fragrance is used to induce sleep, overcome frigidity and to facilitate childbirth. The form generally used is oil of jasmine, available at Kiehl's.

JELLY BAG: A flannel or cotton bag used to strain juice for jellies, etc.

KEROSENE OIL: Kerosene.

LANOLIN: A grease refined from wool, used in cosmetics and medicinal preparations. Available at your drugstore where it is called "toilet lanolin."

LAUREL LEAVES: Now commonly available on your grocery store shelves as bay leaves.

MACE: The caul (covering) of the nutmeg. It is used as a flavoring in cooking and as a carminative in medicinal preparations.

MACERATE: To extract the flavor or useful properties of a substance by steeping in a liquid.

MALAGA RAISINS: Unusually sweet raisins grown in Spain. Substitute good-quality raisins.

MALLOW: A plant with much mucilage in the stalks and leaves which are used as a soothing dressing for burns and skin irritations, and as the basis for many sore throat and cold remedies. This mucilage is also the basis for making marshmallows.

MARJORAM: An herb used in cooking and some medicinal and cosmetic preparations.

MARROW: The pulpy matter found inside most bones, specifically large beef bones. It is used in cooking and in certain cosmetic preparations.

MINK OIL: Oil derived from mink, valued for its extreme emolliency. Available from Caswell-Massey.

MINT: Also called spearmint. It is used in potpourris, medicinal preparations, and cooking.

MUSHROOM KETCHUP: A condiment made from mushrooms, very popular in colonial times. Still available at specialty shops.

MUSK: Obtained from glands found on the male musk deer. It is used in some medicinal preparations, but its main use is as a fixative in perfumes and potpourris. Since the musk deer is facing extinction, please buy synthetic Musk which is just as effective as the real thing. Available from Caswell-Massey.

MYRRH: The resin of the tree that resembles a cedar. It is used in incense, perfumes, medicinal preparations, and cosmetics.

NUTMEG: The fruit of an evergreen tree grown in the Molucca Islands. It is used as a perfume in cosmetics, in cooking as a flavoring, and medicinally to promote digestion, stop vomiting, and as a stimulant.

OLEUM LINI: Linseed oil.

OLEUM TEREBINTH: Turpentine.

ORANGE FLOWER WATER: A water prepared from orange flowers, much used by the colonials. Available in specialty shops and from Caswell-Massey.

ORRIS: The dried root of the Florentine iris. It is used as a fixative in potpourris, and in tooth powders and some cosmetics.

PALM OIL: The oil derived from the fruit of the palm tree, much used in cosmetics.

PARSLEY: A common herb that contains large amounts of vitamins A & C, and is rich in the minerals iron, iodine, copper and manganese. It is much used in cooking, and very occasionally in medicinal preparations.

PECTORAL: A preparation used to treat maladies of the respiratory tract.

PENNYROYAL: A member of the mint family. It is an excellent insect repellent, and is used medicinally as a diuretic.

PERSIC OIL: Oil obtained from apricot kernels; apricot oil.

PORTER: A type of weak sweet stout.

POTPOURRI: A scented preparation made from flower petals, herbs, spices and other aromatic substances used to perfume rooms, clothes, etc.

PROOF SPIRIT: 100-proof alcohol.

RAISIN WINE: A sweet white dessert wine; Muscatel.

ROSEMARY: An aromatic herb much used in cooking, cosmetics, and medicinal preparations.

SAFFRON: The petals from the flowers of the crocus family, used mainly as a yellow coloring in cooking and for its slight flavor.

SAGE: A common herb used in cooking, cosmetics, and medicinal preparations.

SALERATUS: The colonial equivalent of baking powder.

SARASPIRILLA (also SARSAPARILLA): A South American vine much prized for its medicinal qualities.

SASSAFRAS: A tree native to North America. Bark and roots are used medicinally as a blood purifier, diaphoretic, diuretic, and for inflammations of the joints. Chewing the bark is said to decrease one's desire for tobacco.

SEVILLE ORANGE: A type of Spanish orange much used for marmalades and colonial cooking. Any thin-skinned orange will do as a substitute.

SHALLOT: A member of the onion family with a flavor between onions and garlic.

STORAX: Also called Styrax or Sterax. Obtained from the sap of four types of trees of which witch hazel is one. It has the same action as benzoin.

SWEET BAGS: Small cloth bags filled with sweet-scented herbal preparations to induce sleep, scent clothes, etc.

TARRAGON: An herb used extensively in cooking.

THYME: A common herb of the mint family. It is used in cooking and in medicinal preparations as a stimulant, antiseptic, anesthetic for the mucous membranes, and as a rub for muscular aches and pains.

TINCTURE: An alcoholic solution containing medicinal substances.

TREACLE: An old term for molasses.

VETIVER: An aromatic grass with a sandalwood-like fragrance. It is used for its scent and also as an excellent fixative.

WITCH HAZEL: A shrub native to the eastern United States. The bark is brewed into a liquid much used as an astringent and tonic.

Colonial measures are confusing to today's cook, so I've compiled the following table.

COLONIAL MEASURE	MODERN EQUIVALENT
1 pennyweight	1/20 ounce
1 drachm	1/8 ounce
1 small pinch	1/16 teaspoon
1 large pinch	1/8 teaspoon
1 saltspoon	1/4 teaspoon
3 teaspoons	1 tablespoon
1 dessertspoon	2 teaspoons
1 small coffee cup	3/4 cup
1 large teacup	1 cup
1 small teacup	1/2 cup
1 wineglass	1/4 cup
1 tumbler	1 cup
1 gill	1/2 cup
1 ounce allspice, powdered	4½ tablespoons
1 ounce almond extract	2 tablespoons
1 ounce cinnamon, powdered	4½ tablespoons
1 ounce cloves, powdered	4 tablespoons
1 ounce mustard, powdered	4½ tablespoons
1 ounce nutmeg, powdered	3½ tablespoons
1 ounce pepper, ground	3½ tablespoons
1 pint of raw eggs	10 eggs
1 pint of egg whites	18 egg whites
1 pint of egg yolks	24 egg yolks
Butter the size of a filbert	1 rounded teaspoon
Butter the size of a hazelnut	1 rounded teaspoon
Butter the size of a butternut	1 rounded dessertspoon
Butter the size of a walnut	1 rounded tablespoon
Butter the size of a hen's egg	2 ounces

Colonial receipts call for all sorts of sugar we're not familiar with—loaf sugar, double-refined loaf sugar, moist sugar, powdered loaf sugar—none of them available today. Substitute regular granulated sugar by adding half of what the receipt requires, tasting, then adding more until it's sweetened to your taste.

Where to Find & Buy Ingredients

The following are mail-order companies I've dealt with that carry the herbs, oils, and other ingredients you'll need in order to use these receipts. Please send them a note first asking how much they charge for their catalogs—it's difficult to stay in business if they have to send out free catalogs to everyone who requests one.

CASWELL-MASSEY
MAIL-ORDER DEPT.
320 West 13th Street
New York, New York 10014
Tel. (212) 675-2210

CASWELL-MASSEY
RETAIL STORE
518 Lexington Avenue
   at 48th Street
New York, New York 10017

A catalog from Caswell-Massey is a pleasure for anyone, whether or not you're in search of ingredients for these receipts! They are my #1 favorite pharmacy—established in 1752 and supplying colognes, soaps, essential oils, ingredients for making potpourris, and exotic